Further praise for *A Barefoot Doctor's Guide for Women*

"Having experienced the throes of the menopause of two women, I breathed a sigh of relief at the possibility of some help. And yet, this book is not only useful for health issues unique to women. We all are subject to the growing pollution of the body by the environment, food, antibiotics, and stress. Dr. Georgette Delvaux gives clear and intelligent advice on how to deal with widespread problems of inflammation, indigestion, fluid retention, and a host of other challenges facing us as we age."

—**Don Hanlon Johnson, PhD**, Professor of
Somatics, California Institute of Integral Studies
and author of *Everyday Hopes, Utopian Dreams*

"In her new book, *A Barefoot Doctor's Guide for Women,* Georgette Delvaux, DC, leads us on a delightful and informative romp through the female body, mind, and spirit. With her light, informal but informed tone, she addresses such troubling issues as premenstrual syndrome, menopause and hot flashes, breast care, fibroid tumors, osteoporosis, hip fracture, nutrition, dehydration, insomnia, and anxiety. In each case she gives us useful, practical information about the condition, describes the Western medical approach to treatment, and then suggests several natural, complementary approaches as alternative treatments for the same condition. For each treatment she presents both the advantages and the disadvantages, but it seems clear that her personal and professional preference is for the 'Barefoot Doctor's' approach. By the time you finish reading the last page, you may find yourself reconsidering your own choices for the health and well-being of your body, mind, and spirit."

— **Sandy Dibbel-Hope, PhD**, Clinical Psychologist

"Dr. Georgette Delvaux is a healer. Her special talent is her ability to integrate the best wisdom and skills from all healing arts, beyond the definitions of 'Eastern' and 'Western,' and to arrive at an integrated paradigm for understanding our bodies. Her book helps us understand our natural rhythms, seasons, and changes so that we know intuitively when we are well, when we are ill, when our changes are alarm bells, and when they are natural progressions of our life seasons. Dr. Delvaux shares with us her understanding of our bodies' ability to weather changes and our innate ability to heal ourselves."
— **LizHendrickson, JD**

"Though written as a medical tour guide for women, Georgette Delvaux's book transformed my attitude toward the female body. Along with awe toward its inestimable power to seduce and reproduce, I now see a central place for gentleness, kindness, and care toward its natural vulnerability."
—**Karl Kracklauer, PhD**

A BAREFOOT DOCTOR'S
guide *for* women

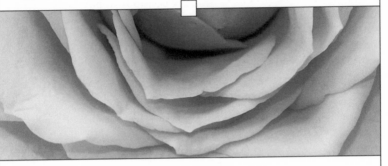

· tales about well-being ·

for my patients, my colleagues, my friends, and all women

georgette maria delvaux

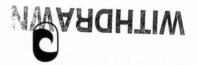
North Atlantic Books
Berkeley, California

Published by
North Atlantic Books
P.O. Box 12327
Berkeley, California 94712

Cover and book design by Maxine Ressler
Cover photo © Jasmin Awad/iStockphoto.com
Printed in the United States of America

A Barefoot Doctor's Guide for Women is sponsored by the Society for the Study of Native Arts and Sciences, a nonprofit educational corporation whose goals are to develop an educational and crosscultural perspective linking various scientific, social, and artistic fields; to nurture a holistic view of arts, sciences, humanities, and healing; and to publish and distribute literature on the relationship of mind, body, and nature.

North Atlantic Books' publications are available through most bookstores. For further information, call 800-337-2665 or visit our website at www.northatlanticbooks.com.

Substantial discounts on bulk quantities are available to corporations, professional associations, and other organizations. For details and discount information, contact our special sales department.

LIBRARY OF CONGRESS CATALOGING-IN-PUBLICATION DATA

Delvaux, Georgette Maria.
    A barefoot doctor's guide for women / by Georgette Maria Delvaux.
        p. cm.
    Summary: "Providing an integrated, commonsense approach to women's hormonal health, this book brings together materials from diverse sources—alternative and conventional medical journals, acupuncture, homeopathy, naturopathy, and the personal experience of the author and her patients—into a single resource"—Provided by publisher.
    Includes index.
        ISBN-13: 978-1-55643-665-9
        ISBN-10: 1-55643-665-3
    1. Women—Health and hygiene—Popular works.   2. Women—Diseases—Alternative treatment—Popular works.   3. Endocrine gynecology—Popular works.   4. Hormones—Popular works.   I. Title.
    RA778.D3337 2007
    613'.04244—dc22   2007020148

1 2 3 4 5 6 7 8 9 United 14 13 12 11 10 09 08 07

To Michael Salveson,
my Man for All Seasons

acknowledgments

I THANK MY Rolfing teachers, Michael Salveson, Peter Melchior, and Jan Sultan for showing me that the first step to helping someone is observation without preconception.

I thank my friend and acupuncturist Margaret Arent, MAc, DiplAc, CA, for being the guardian of my health.

I thank my homeopath, Ellen Gunther, MD, for showing me the difference between hormonal surges and emotional fragility.

I thank Clara Felix, PhD, for being a brilliant and irreverent nutritionist and unflappable in the face of bogus, vitamin-bashing research. I thank Paulina Warren, PhD, for helping me clearly understand how our food can either support or damage our vitality.

I thank Nancy Gardner, PhD, for introducing me to Thermography. I thank Joan J. McKenna, PhD, for showing me the insidious process of fluid retention.

I thank my patients for letting me gawk at them and pester them about the details of their lives.

I thank my grandmothers, aunts, and female relatives for being oblivious to the presence of an eavesdropping little girl who listened, mouth open, to their woes, who observed their mistakes and sad self-deceptions, and who kept thinking that there must be a different way.

I thank my first editor, Caroline Knapp for, oh so carefully, pushing a little here and pulling a little there until I made the book I wanted to make: short, easy to read, and easy to understand.

Un homme prévenu en vaut deux,
une femme prévenue en vaut dix.

A forewarned man is worth two,
a forewarned woman is worth ten.

—FRENCH PROVERB

preamble

FOR WHOM EXACTLY are you writing this book, asked my friends when I began writing. I had trouble answering. It seemed obvious to me that many people would be interested in the information you'll find here—every woman, for certain, any practitioner, man or woman, who does not have extensive medical training and works with women. Adult men who know or like or spend any time at all with women might be curious about these themes for their own sake. Isn't that almost everybody, if we leave out, obviously, those who already know all of this, and give a wide berth to misogynists, inveterate bachelors, and misguided people. Last but not least, we would excuse hermits, of course.

Not that the information presented below is new. All of it can be found somewhere else and in much more detail, if you take the time to search for it. My purpose is to bring the important pieces of information together in one place. I'll speak about the delicate balance of a woman's health, to show how and when it can shift out of phase, how to restore it before any damage has occurred, and when to start looking for help if damage is developing.

table of contents

introduction

DURING THE CULTURAL Revolution (1966–1974) of the Mao Tse-Tung years in China, medical care collapsed. Doctors trained in the medicine of the West were accused of being influenced by capitalism, and many were killed or jailed as traitors. Furthermore, all intelligent and educated people were suspicious *per se* if they voiced opinions that did not coincide with the reigning doctrine. Most doctors fled the country or went underground. This resulted in the loss of about three-quarters of the country's medical practitioners. Alarmed by this situation, the authorities decided to train as many young people as possible in the most basic traditional Chinese medicine. These young people were called "barefoot doctors." They were trained in the bare minimum of traditional acupuncture and manual therapy, they knew basic midwifery, they could set broken bones, etc. They lived among the common folk, the poorest of the poor, the farm and factory workers. They had strictly nothing to work with but their hands, their acupuncture needles, and their knowledge, and I am sure that some of them were barefoot. I see them as the guerrilleros of health care; my Taoist teacher called them "a godsend beyond godsend."

How much they must have relied on their powers of observation! And yet we all can simply see or feel a multitude of signs that tell us about health: skin color and dryness; vitality of hair and nails; sclera of the eye; swollen, cavernous, or discolored eye sockets; quality of pulse and breathing rhythm; body alignment;

swelling of joints and elasticity of joint motion; muscle tone and range of motion; smell of breath and sweat; variations of girth that tell us about habits, excesses or deficiencies, peristaltic sounds that tell us about the state of the autonomic nervous system, just to name the most obvious. For less noticeable factors, a few simple questions can often tell us a great deal about the location, quality, and timing of pain. We can ask about changes as the day passes; about when fatigue or pain sets in and after what kind of activity and how much of it. In the past, these warning signs guided all health professionals. There is no reason to abandon them now that extremely sophisticated imaging procedures and laboratory tests have been developed. The modern tools are expensive and are most useful for rescuing those who are in danger. Even with no actual medical training, anyone who is interested and observant can notice trouble of many kinds and would instinctively be highly alarmed upon seeing a person who, for instance, was extremely pale, sweated profusely, and had labored breathing.

It may be that my colleagues, the practitioners of manual medicine, can help with only some of what they observe or find out through these methods. However, that fact does not mean for them to ignore observations that indicate trouble and might be helped by others. In particular, body workers often feel that it is not their place to speak to their female patients about women's health problems that they observe or suspect. Women body workers, however, have an advantage: We are in the same boat as our female patients. Women will answer questions about their reproductive health if we care to ask them.

There are more women than ever before practicing manual medicine, as Rolfers, chiropractors, Pilates trainers, and osteopaths, to name just a few. Some of these women have "women's troubles" themselves. The formerly taboo topic of women's health is entering mainstream awareness simply because there are more of us who are interested in understanding and changing it. My teacher and friend Jan Sultan, a senior faculty member of the Rolf Institute, recently said to me, with astonished raised eyebrows: "I can't believe how many women I am training lately, and I can't believe how good they are at this. I think that in the future women are going to take over the entire medical profession. And that is a good thing."

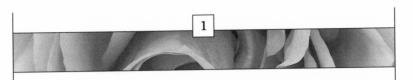

premenstrual syndrome

*Yogis should be examples, I struggled hard, and
many people may be having the same feelings I was
undergoing. So why should I not give out so they
know the truth, so they also get the courage?*
—B. K. S. IYENGAR

IN THE WORLD of medicine, a syndrome is an aggregate of signs
and symptoms which, taken together, form the picture of a
disease. The origin of this word is Greek; it means "a running
together, a tumultuous concourse." Regarding premenstrual
syndrome we truly are on a tumultuous concourse, unless we
agree with Roseanne Barr that "Women complain about premenstrual syndrome, but I think of it as the only time of the
month when I can be myself."

The premenstrual phase of the menstrual cycle usually starts at
ovulation, two weeks after onset of the menses. It can announce
itself with a temporary minor pain in an ovary, the so-called
Mittelschmerz, a German word meaning "pain in the middle of the
cycle." This pain accompanies the release of the ovoid from the
follicle, as a little bubble of fluid bursts and the ovoid makes its
way down the fallopian tube. Women who experience this pain
often don't identify what they are feeling, as it can be a very small
sensation. Others feel it clearly.

Women who suffer from premenstrual syndrome almost
immediately feel a "drop" in their mood after ovulation. Then

a gradual buildup of peripheral fluid follows. The breasts swell and hurt. The abdomen and often the legs swell, more so at the end of the day. The eyes look puffy in the morning. Gradual constipation can set in because fluids are not released into the large intestine. A first vague, then growing, sense that one's beloved has become really insensitive is not uncommon. Nor is accidentally breaking dishes or patiently waiting for the light to turn green while merely stopped at a stop sign.

As soon as menstrual bleeding starts, the dark mood lifts, and then, like magic, with frequent urination and restarting of normal bowel regularity, the swelling goes away. That's when British women say, "I've got the curse," and the French whisper, "Les Anglais ont débarqué" (that is, "the English have disembarked," a reference to the bloody territorial invasions with which the French and English aristocrats entertained each other in past centuries).

When I complained about the extreme ups and downs of my cycle, my well-meaning homeopath told me, "It is because you are a woman." I insisted that it did not feel right, to which he countered, "It is because you are that much of a woman!" and gave me a remedy for being a pansy (I looked it up). What a nice way to state your ignorance!

For the more innovative orthomolecular doctors, also called naturopaths, these bad hair weeks are classified as episodes of "endocrine disruption." In this case the disruption is an excess of estrogen and a deficiency of progesterone—more specifically, a lack of progesterone at the moment the ovoid is released. If nothing is done about this imbalance it will persist and may develop into more serious problems as menopause approaches. For a woman who enters menopause with an existing hormone imbalance, it will certainly be a very disruptive ride. It may impair her judgment and endanger her health, particularly if she feels unwell enough to quickly agree to the still-common practice of taking artificial hormones. Artificial hormones almost always get rid of all symptoms in a very short time, but they leave women exposed to potential trouble later.

Recently, newspapers have been full of articles about the pros and cons of artificial hormone supplementation, which until 2002 was advocated as a safe and necessary routine for all women.[1] The Nurses Health Study, a large observational study in the 1970s, started an ongoing debate and launched many large and small studies regarding hormone supplementation.[2] Still, most people don't know that the hormones used in these studies are not bio-identical hormones (which are hormones exactly like ours but extracted from plants), and that they have dangerous side effects just because they are artificial hormones (which are hormones *almost* exactly like ours but partly synthetic). At this point, doctors are not anywhere near a consensus on how to proceed with hormone supplementation.

Let's have a look at a scientific theory about estrogen excess, one which no doubt is familiar to many of you already. According to this theory, estrogen becomes dominant in our bodies because most environmental pollutants—artificial hormones fed to the animals whose meat we eat, pesticides in our fruits and vegetables, industrial pollutants and plastics entering our food chain and our bodies through accidental exposure or blatant neglect—are all structurally similar to our own estrogens, to the extent that our bodies are unable to distinguish these xeno-estrogens (from the Greek *xeno,* meaning "foreign") from our own. The xeno-estrogens are also designed to be structurally much more stable, with far longer half-lives than human hormones. Unlike our own more labile estrogens, which disintegrate as soon as they are no longer needed, xeno-estrogens continue to circulate in our bodies for a long time. Their presence is said to cause the premenstrual symptoms described above—and worse.

These estrogen-dominant conditions can be serious enough

to become scandalous! In men excessive estrogen from food can cause swelling of the mammary glands. In children, shockingly premature sexual development can appear in extreme instances. Cases of ovarian and uterine cancers have been seen in eight-year-old girls who also have breasts and pubic hair, and testicular cancer has been seen in young boys with fully developed sexual organs. In the early stages of the imbalance, women tend to gain weight, without overeating. In fact, their bodies are not really invested with fat; what makes them heavy is fluid retention.

A telling anecdote: My husband and I wanted to have a late dinner in a new restaurant and chatted with the chef to have him agree to cook for us, even though he was already closing up. We spoke about red meat and how to make sure that it is of good quality. I found out from that chef that meat raised with hormones looks very good at first but when cooked, it oozes water and the meat becomes dry and hard. I know, this is a very crude analogy; please don't hold it against me.

Preservatives are another potentially harmful category of substances with an estrogen-like activity, one that is ubiquitous in prepared foods and in cosmetics.[3] Let's look at one kind among the many: parabens. They are found in cosmetics and are thought to be specifically damaging to breast cells. They are used in antiperspirants, deodorants, creams, lotions, liquid soaps, shampoos, lipsticks, and more. Read the labels! They are called ethylparaben, methylparaben, butylparaben, and they also appear combined, as in ethylbutylparaben. They are often fraudulently listed simply as "fragrance." You find them everywhere in conventional cosmetics, as well as in so-called "all natural" cosmetics.

I lost my patience with one particular aggressively advertised skin cream, which touted a long list of doctors of all sorts who had consulted in the manufacturing of their marvelous, high-vitamin and high-antioxidant product. I asked them about the estrogen-like parabens which I saw in the list of its ingredients. One of their doctors answered me in writing that no research existed that showed parabens causing damage to human tissue. This is what is usually said, and it is technically quite true. There is no research that shows that parabens cause damage to human tissue. But what kind of research has been done? And for how long? Was this research done on rabbits? On rats? In vitro human tissue? To prove his point this doctor magnanimously told me that he himself is using the product. How silly! He's a man! He does not use multiple cosmetics as many women do, and he does not have monthly cycles. Any ill effect caused by parabens would most likely remain below the threshold of his perception, and it certainly would not present itself as a monthly imbalance—even though I wished it on him for half a minute!

Parabens are only a few in a long list of ingredients present in cosmetics that are now being found to have undesirable, hormone-like effects on us. Think about how many cosmetics you use in a day, how many times a day, and for how many years? Wouldn't it make sense that the effects of even a minimally damaging substance would gradually accumulate? So, what did I do? I took myself and my magnifying glasses to my favorite New Age pharmacy. I spent several hours perusing long lists of ingredients, looking for the absence of parabens. I ended up attracting the attention of the clerks, who dutifully helped me. I did find one or two products that use citrus extracts and vitamin C as preservatives. Then I went home and, in a huff, threw away my entire battery of look-good and feel-good treasures.

I am not saying that all of women's hormone-related problems are due solely to environmental, household, and cosmetic pollution. I would like that to be true because I think a problem of that kind can be remedied with awareness and knowledge. Hormone imbalance, however, like all other health problems, has always existed to some extent. In the nineteenth century these problems had nonspecific names like neurasthenia (chronic mental and physical fatigue). Laudanum was then recommended. Laudanum was made from opium: the pharmacologists thought they had found a non-addictive opiate. Of course it wasn't. Women who used laudanum became addicted.

Like any other disease, hormone imbalance may be due to the stresses we expose ourselves to and to the effect of cumulative mistakes we make, like smoking, drinking, dieting, overeating, taking drugs, and not resting. The part of our body that is the most fragile is the part that will become ill first. It may be that most diseases are due to simple aging, to genetic damage, or to bad luck. Specific women's problems may, of course, also have all these possible causes.

It's important to remember, in the midst of all this confusion about causes, that many of these problems are treatable, especially when they are identified early. Let's take an example: A hormone imbalance can happen to a very young woman. If it is not treated it will persist throughout her life. In the early stages she may not feel well but she also may not be able even to think that something is wrong. She is always unhappy and tired, she has a swollen belly, she finds anything that happens such a drag, and she dreads her period. At this stage the problem is not that difficult to treat and cure. It needs to be recognized first and then examined from different points of view. What is out of balance? The hormones? The thyroid? The adrenals? The diet? Other factors? The only safe approach would be to go to a health practitioner and let him or her take the case. An acupuncturist, an Ayurvedic practitioner, or an herbalist would probably advise very specific herbs and vitamins; naturopaths would do a good study of lab values, and if hormones were needed they would prescribe bio-identical hormones, monitor the progress of the recovery, and stop the supplementation soon after balance was achieved. We saw that "bio-identical" means "the same as life."

The hormones administered need to be exactly what is missing, and they need to originate from plants and not from mares. I really did write "mares"—female horses, yes! Conventional artificial estrogen prescribed for women is extracted from pregnant mare urine. Neigh at it! These prescriptions do contain what is needed, but they also contain other charming horse hormones that might make you very attractive to nice rowdy stallions.

pain during
the menstrual cycle

CAN PAIN EVER be called "normal"? When does a strong sensation become pain? Pain indicates a problem. It is not a sign. It is a symptom. A sign, like blood pressure or elevated temperature, can be observed and measured by anybody. A symptom is experienced by the patient; it is what the person tells you. She can give you a description, for example: "From one to ten, ten being the worst pain I ever felt, this feels like it is a five." This tells you about how troubled the person feels, but it does not give you any objective information.

Pain at ovulation in the area of an ovary, the *Mittelschmerz* I described above, should be short and is generally thought of as mild. Pain deeply behind the pubic area just prior to or with the beginning of menstruation can be slightly spasm-like and is indicative of the cervix expanding to let the blood flow through. It may be strong but should also be short, lasting not more than several hours.[*]

Pain in the lower back, lumbar spine and/or the sacrum that only happens before and around menstruation almost certainly indicates that there is an abnormal side-to-side pull or rotation between the sacrum and the utero-sacral ligaments. The uterus is well attached in the pelvis by its ligamentous moorings. Its correct position is central, really central. The uterus and its attachments create a transverse structure, not unlike that of the diaphragm, and they literally hold the lower part of the small intestines up and in place. An unevenly located uterus will exert an uneven pull on the sacrum and vice versa, via the utero-sacral ligaments. Other structures can be involved: sacro-iliac joints, pubic symphysis, piriformis, ilio-sacral ligaments, ilio-lumbar ligaments, the joints of the lumbar vertebrae, the quadratus lumborum, the ligaments of the bladder, etc.

This type of back pain is not really considered worthy of medical attention beyond the advice to take an aspirin. It is true that this pain is transitory... in the beginning. But it is due to a structural imbalance; the anatomy has slipped from its good position. If the imbalance is not corrected it will persist and get worse, causing increasing pain, and eventually it will create inflammation and arthritic changes in the joints. A good osteopath or a good Rolfer can help.

Any other type of pain may need medical attention. Constant pain that gets gradually worse, becomes disabling before menstruation, and is accompanied by very heavy bleeding can indicate serious trouble, the least of which could be endometriosis. This word means "too much uterine lining." Like many of the problems related to the female reproductive cycle, it is thought to be caused by an excess of estrogen combined with a deficiency of progesterone. In endometriosis the inside layer of the cells of the uterus develops beyond the uterus and grows via the fallopian tubes into the abdominal cavity. As menstruation approaches this misplaced intra-uterine tissue swells just like the lining of the uterine walls, building a milieu that could, in theory, receive a fertilized ovum. The process causes serious pain, cramping, and excessive bleeding. A young woman with this predicament will barely be able to conceive. If she does conceive, there is an increased risk that the embryo will implant itself in the tissue outside the uterus. This is called extra-uterine pregnancy and is life-threatening to the woman.

As far as I know there is no treatment available for endometriosis other than artificial hormone therapies that have a great variation of adverse effects and/or surgery. The surgery removes the abnormally proliferated tissue. That is generally the extent of the treatment. If the hormone imbalance persists, the problem will come back soon. The doctors know that the problem will most probably come back, and they advise the patient to try to become pregnant within several months after the surgery or else the new proliferation of tissue will again prevent pregnancy. The only permanent conventional treatment for endometriosis is the surgical removal of the ovaries, with resulting infertility and early menopause.

A better approach might be to consult a naturopathic doctor who would order thorough lab studies of hormone imbalance, prescribe the missing bio-identical hormones, check and recheck until the imbalance is corrected, and, above all, he would teach the young woman how to avoid exposure to xeno-estrogens.

Other problems like very short cycles, two or more menstruations a month, excessive bleeding (loosely defined as soaking two or more menstrual pads per hour for more than one day), skipped menstruations, or no menstruation at all for many months are all indications of serious trouble, and a gynecologist must be consulted.

The good news is that most often even serious trouble can be completely remedied if it is discovered in its early stages. The debate about what is "normal" should never end. If you do not feel well you are not well and you need to seek advice. Longevity depends not only on good luck but also on good proprioception, the ability to perceive yourself.

proprioception is the sixth sense

WE HAVE FIVE organs of perception, five senses: sight, hearing, smell, touch, and taste. How strange that proprioception, the sensing of our own body, is not on the list. Technically proprioception is the sensory feedback that we get from our skin, our muscles, and joints; it is also called the position sense. It constantly lets us know where our limbs are, and how the body is positioned in space. This sense is supposedly not conscious. We do not think of every motion we do when we walk up a flight of stairs, for example—we may actually make it up the stairs thinking of something completely different or doing something else at the same time, like carrying a tray of food. We also constantly adapt parts of our body unconsciously to movements we do consciously. For example: let's suppose we are standing up and we are going to lift an arm. Before we move the arm at all, we will unconsciously contract a deep calf muscle (soleus) in both legs to stabilize ourselves. If this did not happen the weight of the lifting arm would make us lose our balance, and we would be pretty graceless, even clumsy. You can really see the crucial importance of this ability of our brain when it is not there anymore. Observe stroke patients who have lost this ability. If they are lucky enough to be able to walk at all, they have to look at what their legs are doing; they have to constantly command their movements consciously or else they cannot move correctly. If one leg is affected, for example, and they look somewhere else as they walk, that leg will just drag along and they will fall. If simply standing, they would fall down in case of a power failure—surprised by darkness, unable to see, and therefore unable to control their movements.

That is the traditional medical way of understanding proprioception. The roots of this word mean "perceiving of self." I am so sorry that perceiving such an important part of ourselves has been relegated to the unconscious. Let's not leave it there anymore.

Dr. Ida Rolf, who created Rolfing, had a legendary ability to perceive what was happening to someone's body without touching. When she asked my teacher to become a teacher he realized that he needed to understand how she was able to perceive so accurately. He arranged to sit beside her while she was teaching. He noticed that, as she observed the patient, she would suddenly become quiet, her body would fully relax, and it seemed like her attention was completely focused inward. Then she would make an accurate observation that would befuddle everyone. After watching Dr. Rolf do this a few times he realized that she was observing subtle reactions in herself that were responses to what was happening in the person she was observing. That was when he understood how he too could use his subtle sense of self to get information about his patients.

We can all learn to become more aware of what we feel. We all can learn the significance of what our proprioception tells us. Rolfing, Osteopathy, Homeopathy, the Feldenkrais and Alexander techniques, Pilates and Gyrotonic, Yoga and Martial Arts (Chi Gung, Tai Chi, Capoeira, Jiu Jitsu, Tai Qwon Do, etc.), and even good dance training—whether these practices are done to us or we learn from a teacher, they all work on a similar level: they heal and refine our self-sensing. Not only the sensing of where our body is in space and how it moves, they sharpen all senses that relate to motion and well-being. These abilities are not only the result of inborn talent; they rely on motivation and training. Considering what a master of martial arts can do and what a diligent student can learn from her, it seems to me that proprioception and conscious motion are not that clearly separated. Furthermore, there is no time in the life of a person when this ability cannot be cultivated anymore, unless the nervous tissue is totally destroyed. Even serious scarring should not be a reason to despair. Very old people, if they take up careful treatment and training, can rehabilitate damaged areas. The damaged areas could be joints, muscles, ligaments, and inner organs.

Teachers and practitioners of any fine manual healing art have exquisitely sensitive hands. They are able to feel deeply into the body of people when they diagnose and treat. They only look like they use just their hands! What they really do is feel with their entire body, they "melt" with the patient's body, they relax their hands and body to a degree that information is picked up by their hand, the lower arm, the elbow, the upper arm, their eyes, their nose, their ears, etc. They are also keen observers and they use all techniques of direct observation and interrogation that I have mentioned before, like skin color, smell, pulse, psychological disposition, etc.

And here comes my point: This perception, in order to be useful, must include the willingness to take oneself seriously, to trust that what one senses and feels is real, to really accept the information our proprioception gives us. Most of us have been conditioned to trust teachers, preachers, parents, and assorted "big" people more than ourselves, and as a result many people are severely critical of themselves and their abilities. In the words of John Upledger, DO, teacher of Osteopathy: "... the potential of humankind is limited only by its own concept of that limitation."

People can feel minor trouble starting in their own bodies.

We all have the faculty of proprioception. Some of us have had more training and may be able to know more about what we feel. Some of us, however, decide that a minor chronic pain should be considered normal aging and ignored. Let's take the example of the pain of excessive stomach acidity. It can be due to a number of reasons ranging from too much acid food or alcohol to too much stress and anxiety. Taking an over-the-counter antacid takes care of the problem. It really does. Every time. But not for long. The problem recurs if the causes remain. Some people let this go until they have an ulcer . . . an open wound inside their stomach! If you speak to them about it they most probably will remember when it started, how long it has been troubling them, for how long the pain has been strong, and for how long they have been ignoring it. If you feel that you have a problem, don't start by minimizing the information coming from your senses. Accept the information as reality, particularly if you don't know what the message is. You cannot change what you don't notice; you cannot notice what you don't accept.

A word of caution: There are extensive resources of information about health care freely available on the Internet, in publications, in health food stores, in encyclopedias. Only use these resources to help yourself understand. As we have seen in the case of stomach acidity, self-help is a double-edged sword. It is tempting to associate a symptom with a remedy; the advertising industry has us well indoctrinated. Just consider how much the do-it-yourself craze has developed the hardware business. I myself have succumbed and done repair jobs, just because I thought there was nothing to it. I learned how steep the learning curve for becoming a handy (wo)man is, and that lesson cost me a fair amount of money.

In the face of a medical problem the consequences of self-help could not only affect your purse. Even gathering information by yourself can lead you astray. Taking any substances—herbs and particularly hormones—even if they are natural, bio-identical, plant-derived, low dose, etc., can hurt you and even confuse a practitioner who is trying to take care of you. But you will be a better patient if you give a true and detailed report about what is happening to you. It seems to me that the very first step toward healing must start with affectionate self-respect. Respect and honor what you feel! Even Jesus recommended that we should love other people "like we love ourselves." When His Holiness the Dalai Lama was first introduced to the concept of self-hatred he thought that his translator had made an unfortunate mistake.

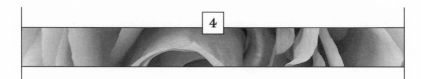

menopause

In PAST CENTURIES most women spent their fertile years being pregnant, nursing their babies, and attending to their children, their husband, and their household. Only in rare cases would they have been able to attend to any personal affairs like careers, artistic talents, or other ambitions and callings. When the time for menopause came many women, due to problems similar to those described in this book, lost their interest in intercourse and, as a consequence, also lost their intimate relationship with their husband, though not necessarily their friendship and respect. Common opinion considered it wise to overlook or tolerate mistresses as long as they stayed "in their place."

An interesting aside: It has been observed that the women of simpler cultures (for example, in places like rural Africa and rural India) have more pregnancies and not as many breast cancers or uterine cancers. This is attributed to the fact that they do not "force" their reproductive organs to not reproduce, as women often do in the Western world. This point of view implies that the constant monthly periods of otherwise healthy women who do not have children end up creating monthly hormonal roller coasters, so to speak, that facilitate the development of cancers in the later years. Many gynecologists believe that it is to a woman's advantage to use her reproductive organs at least once. They think that a woman's never having taken her body through a pregnancy is a risk factor. I will add my little grain of salt to this by asserting that contraception via artificial hormones is certainly a risky way to avoid pregnancy.

What I just told you does not mean that all is well for the health of women from Africa or India, who can give birth to eight or ten children during their reproductive years, including a few miscarriages. Except for their tribal midwives, these women do not have any health care. The multiple births, often starting at a very young age when their bodies are not fully grown, can cause deep lacerations to their pelvic floor. The really unlucky ones can end up with prolapsed organs or a damaged pelvic floor that does not heal. It can leave them permanently incontinent, which results in their certain exclusion from their communities for being unclean.

Menopause in our so-called civilized countries has unfortunately become a cause for intense anxiety and fearful anticipation. The general belief is that your tissues will sag, your wrinkles will deepen, your vagina will dry up, your beauty will vanish, your "nerves will be frayed," you will become hard to live with, and your partner will lose interest and turn his or her desires to younger women.

Relationships often do fail during this time. But probably not only because of what is happening to women. Let's not forget that something called andropause can start happening to men in their sixties, and it too can cause physical and psychological trouble. It is only whispered about, so be discreet. The signs of this could include a brand new expensive red sports car and concurrent excessive or hysterical behavior (oops, does this word ever describe things our men can do?). This, luckily, is not the subject of our discourse.

There is, however, a general consensus among many women that menopause is a blessing and a liberation. The lucky ones who sail through it without much suffering report a beautiful rise in vitality. Margaret Mead, the great anthropologist, is said to have coined the expression "post-menopausal zest." A patient of mine reported that a wonderful black woman from Louisiana had explained to her why many women accomplish great feats only after menopause: "You cain't think straight until your parts stop working!" Women contemplating menopause with dread should stop for a minute to imagine the things they could do with all the energy they invest staying focused and even-minded in the middle of the monthly hormonal fray!

Hormones run our physiology. A look at a basic endocrinology book will make you wonder what in the body is *not* governed by hormones. Premenstrual syndrome is essentially an estrogen/progesterone imbalance that happens when estrogen becomes abnormally dominant. Early menopause is similar: the female reproductive hormones are fading and progesterone diminishes first, which of course comes down to the same thing as having excess estrogen. I would say that minor menopause symptoms look and feel like premenstrual symptoms, in the sense that some of the very chaotic aspects of the first stages of a problematic menopause also present like an excess of estrogen: peripheral fluid retention, intense and chaotic periods, and serious psychological discomfort. The problematic onset of menopause can involve the thyroid gland and the adrenal glands. It may be best to consult a practitioner who will not blindly first prescribe hormones, artificial or bio-identical ones. It may be necessary to consider hormone supplements eventually. If you find yourself at this stage, the moment may have come to reassess your lifestyle, your stress factors, your nutrition, and your nutritional supplements, and to find reliable professional help.

The specific problems caused by peri-menopausal and menopausal hormone imbalances can happen in a number of combinations. Some problems can appear by themselves; often several happen simultaneously. In the conventional medical world they are treated like different problems. They should, of course, be treated when they appear if they have progressed to the point that they interfere with health. The most common conditions are fibrocystic breasts, fibroid tumors of the uterus, osteoporosis and accompanying fractures, dehydration and fluid retention, hot flashes, anxiety, and insomnia. It would be great to have scientific evidence of a connection between these problems, but let's not long for a definitive twenty-year study of thousands of women if we can see what is obvious and hear what women tell us if we care to ask.

fibrocystic breasts and the danger of breast cancer

MANY WOMEN DEVELOP fibrocysts, which are small fibrous cysts or lumps in their breasts, during menopause and in some cases many years before menopause. Breasts can also develop fibroadenomas, which are benign neoplasms, otherwise known as tumors. These can make breasts feel heavy, swollen, inflamed, painful, or lumpy, or all of the above or none of the above. The doctors advise us to have mammograms because they want to be able to detect and monitor these problems and other more dangerous ones. The radiologists carefully examine fibrous tissue: it can look like cancerous tissue though rarely does it really turn out to be cancerous.

Mere uncomplicated fibrocystic breasts are not considered a problem by modern medicine. In the world of dangerous pathology, fibrosis is nothing but neutral connective tissue. Fibrous cysts are considered normal because many women have them. But let's not confuse normal and average here. I do not think that it is normal to have proliferating fibrous tissue in our breasts, even if eighty percent of women over age forty have fibroadenomas.

In a similar vein it is not normal to have arthritis, although almost all people get it. Simple degenerative joint disease, also called osteo-arthritis, with pain, swelling, and reduced and altered joint movement, is due to a pathological inflammatory process caused by the long-term use of joints that are misaligned. This misalignment can result from many different causes: major or minor injuries, overuse, or even simply bad habits. It may be minimal, but if it is not corrected it will end up causing inflammation.

Inflammation, in a nutshell, is a primary response to disease. It precedes and accompanies almost any health problem involving infection or tissue destruction. Chemical change at the site of an open injury, for instance, induces the massive arrival of white blood cells, swelling, and heat. This is inflammation; the word originates in Latin and literally means "incoming flames." The white blood cells destroy bacteria and release substances that form scar tissue, which is tough fibrous tissue.

Inflammation is not in our favor for problems like the joint swelling caused by misalignment, by closed injuries (like blunt trauma and sprains), or by autoimmune diseases like rheumatoid arthritis. Doctors always aim to reduce local inflammation and, in the case of joint problems, for example, recommend rehabilitation as soon as possible to prevent excessive scar formation, which creates a restriction in range of motion. Systematic inflammation tells us that there may be a serious problem developing, like heart damage, autoimmune disease, or malignancy. Decreased inflammation indicates healing. Doctors monitor this with a blood test, the C-Reactive Protein test, which is, or should be, part of all routine annual health exams.

I am going to go way out on a limb now—and I may fall off—but I believe that the fibrous tissue found in the breasts is also the result of an inflammatory process. Fibrocysts and fibroadenomas, which resemble scar tissue in their components, may well be the end stage of constant monthly recurring inflammation caused by excess estrogen and concurrent deficiency of progesterone. We have seen above that this hormonal imbalance, once it has been recognized, can be corrected with bio-identical hormones and hormone-lowering supplements.

The standard medical reaction to any excessive fibrous breast tissue looks something like this: After a routine mammogram, the woman is urged to have a biopsy taken in case the radiologist cannot clearly evaluate a suspicious-looking fibrous area as benign.[5] The pathologist then looks at the biopsied cells under a microscope and sends back a pathology report stating whether or not the suspicious-looking cells from the biopsy are cancerous (a.k.a. malignant). The pathology exam is the only reliable source of information in this matter. The large majority of biopsies, eighty percent, are negative. They nonetheless have nasty side effects: the breast is scarred and may be deformed, and the woman has been thoroughly frightened.

Additional useful diagnostic imaging methods include MRI scans, PET scans, scintimammographies (I promise I did not make this word up), and ultrasounds. Ultrasounds can show if a lump is solid (and most solid tumors are cancerous) or just a benign fluid-filled cyst. All these are very useful and may be recommended in order to gather more information.

A small cancer starts its existence "in situ" ("within the site"), which means that it is inside a capsule or inside a small breast duct (these very small breast cancers are called ductal carcinomas). Ninety-eight percent of these small cancers never do anything. Either they get reabsorbed by the body (as the immune system takes care of them) or they remain there doing nothing, unnoticed. The other two percent of cancers, however, start developing their own blood supply while still "in situ." This process is called neo-angiogenesis (neo = new, angio = blood vessel, genesis = creation). Neo-angiogenesis is what makes an innocent little tumor into a nasty cancer. As soon as a tumor has developed its own blood supply it can grow rapidly. Therefore the argument for recommending early detection via imaging is very sound.

When a cancer is still encapsulated "in situ" it may grow, but as long as it has not spread into the surrounding areas yet it can be removed surgically without risk. However, in my opinion it is not a good idea to break a capsule, to enter and take a biopsy, a small sample of possibly cancerous tissue. If more information is needed—if mammograms, ultrasound and/or scanners point to a problem—the entire little growth should be removed in the first place, as soon as possible and with great care so that the capsule is taken away entirely. This procedure is called lumpectomy. It is dangerous to take just a sample via a needle biopsy or a core biopsy, declare it cancerous, and then spend weeks in palavers weighing lumpectomy versus mastectomy, and chemotherapy versus radiation, and seeking second opinions. There is a chance that cancerous tissue has been liberated by the biopsy and has entered into the blood and the lymphatic system, and that cancerous cells will spread to another part of the body.

The successful removal of an encapsulated lump that is found to have clear margins, i.e., that has no signs of cancerous cells on the outside of the capsule nor in the adjacent lymph nodes, is considered the end of the treatment. The cancer is gone! Chemotherapy is not needed! The fire, so to speak, is extinguished. But have you ever seen the aftermath of a fire in a building? As soon as the smoke has lifted the firefighters take their axes and smash everything in sight that may still be smoldering, and everything that is touching a smoldering remnant. They throw out everything that is a little scorched. And then, of course, the house has to be repaired. Not only the burned parts need to be replaced. The adjacent rooms and even distant areas have been damaged by smoke and are totally unlivable. The entire house needs attention. That is what needs to be done with the body too.

The immune system, the security system of the woman, failed and that was why the tumor developed. Now is the time to figure out what the stress factors were; to look at exposure to carcinogens in the environment, in food, and in cosmetics; and to evaluate the frequency of habitual exhaustion, because all these factors and more can contribute to an immune system breakdown. Then the patient needs to take vitamins, minerals, herbs, essential fatty acids and amino acids. Acupuncture meridians need attention; exercise needs to be reintroduced gradually. In other words the terrain, the biological environment, needs to be restored. Some naturopaths call this "immune system re-education." The entire process can take at least a year or two. If this work does not take place, a weakened and dysfunctional immune system may, once again, fail to perform reliably if cancer cells reappear.

the imaging
of breast tissue

thermography versus mammography,
a complex and most emotional debate

THERMOGRAPHY IS A procedure that records with a computerized imaging system the heat that a substance emits. Recently it has become a new way to study breast tissue. Thermography can indicate a potentially dangerous development in a breast up to ten years before an actual tumor can be found via mammography or skilled palpation.

A thermogram gives us an evaluation of breast tissue via the recording of very subtle temperature differences. The thermographic camera records an image not only of the temperature of the surface of the breasts, but also of the depths of the breast tissue. Thermograms are used in the industrial world, in the military, and in espionage to determine heat variations inside walls or inside buildings, for instance, because heat radiates through matter.

But how can thermography tell us if the heat of breast inflammation is merely due to the hormonal ups and downs of menstruation or menopause, or if it is due to a problem brooding, a tumor that is still in a microscopically small state but that has started to develop and might grow at an explosive rate?

Thermography involves taking two sets of images of the breast temperature. The first one is taken after the patient has spent some time in a cool room with her arms raised, so that the temperature variations caused by clothes and the proximity of the armpits are neutralized. After the first set of heat images has been recorded the patient is asked to cool her hands for a few minutes in icy cold water. This is called "autonomic challenge." The normal response of the sympathetic nervous system (the part of the autonomic nervous system that handles sudden challenges to our inner balance) to this sort of stimulus is to contract blood vessels on the surface. Blood circulation is thus reduced, and the surface of the body cools down in order to maintain normal temperature deep inside. The cold water also cools the temperature of the breasts, which are organs that reside on the surface of the body. But, crucially, this cooling process will not affect the temperature of a developing cancer.

The dreaded process of neo-angiogenesis, the formation of new blood vessels that feed a cancerous tumor, involves nitrous oxide, which is a vasodilator, a substance that forces blood vessels to remain wide open. The scientists who developed breast thermography say that not only do these cancer-feeding blood vessels fail to contract—as normal vessels would—in response to the cooling, they even enlarge!

The genius of thermography shows up when the two sets of images are compared. The overall distribution of temperature looks the same in both thermograms. If no cancer is present the second one shows only a generalized decrease of heat. If there is a problem, the problematic area will "light up" in the second thermogram because the temperature in that area did not cool down—it warmed up. The difference of heat registered can be very small, but the location is clearly visible and measurable to the technician.

Mammography, on the other hand—the most common and still the most widely advocated method of breast screening—happens via X-ray imaging. Let there be no doubt about the fact that X-rays beam ionizing radiation at us, and that any ionizing radiation will damage our DNA, in the tiny amounts used for mammograms or other diagnostic X-rays or in the massive amounts caused by nuclear spills. Moreover, the damage is cumulative. A very small amount of radiation damage, like that caused by a single diagnostic X-ray, may never affect our own lives. Since DNA damage is cumulative, however, our children would risk inheriting our damaged DNA, and so would their children. The chance of descendants somewhere along the line suffering physical consequences from radiation grows as each generation transmits further damaged DNA.

It is true that mammography is not frequently recommended for women of child-bearing age, provided that no problem exists. But problems do exist and what's more, X-rays are ordered in all fields of medicine including dentistry, chiropractic, and podiatry. These days more and more women also attempt to conceive late in life, increasing the chances that they may already have minor DNA damage from other X-rays and from regularly monitoring their breasts via mammograms.

It is reasonable to think that even though non-damaging thresholds of exposure to low-level ionizing radiation do not exist, the benefits of discovering a problem outweigh the risk of damaging the DNA.

I agree that the danger of low exposure to X-rays is preferable to the risk of not discovering a cancer and, of course, DNA does have the ability to repair itself if the immune system is functional. On the other side, why should we submit ourselves and even more, the people coming after us, to potential harm when a very safe routine screening method has become available? Personally, I don't feel so great imagining that more people would have to live with birth defects, which can cause them to remain dependent on others during their entire lives, for the dubious reason that doctors have decided to irradiate women routinely just to find out if they might have a problem.

A further nasty aspect of mammography is the simple brutality of the procedure, as many of us have experienced personally. Is it due to the inexperience or the indifference of some of the technicians, or is it really necessary to compress a breast to a degree that is almost impossible to bear? Women who have breast implants can't even have mammograms because the procedure can rupture the implant. And why do those darn compressing paddles have to be so cold? Another scary fact is that a mammogram performed with excessive pressure can rupture the capsule of an "in-situ" cancerous growth, one still wrapped in its connective tissue, which would mean that cancerous cells would start spreading into the surrounding tissue because of the mammogram.

In spite of all these concerns, mammography remains the most frequently used tool for cancer detection for steadfast traditional doctors. This may be for the simple reason that they either do not know about or do not trust thermography. Most medical professionals I spoke to have no interest in thermography because they do not know about the second set of thermal images that show what the autonomic challenge reveals. It is obvious that without the autonomic challenge a thermograph has very little diagnostic value. I lament the fact that doctors jump to conclusions without knowing the science behind this very useful and safe screening method.

I will take the risk to conclude thus: regular mammograms are not a good way to routinely monitor breast tissue in order to prevent cancer for all the reasons I told you above. A mammogram is very useful, however, for locating an already suspected problem with precision. If the thermogram and the ultrasound and the scanner are indicating trouble, do not refuse a mammogram out of principle. Good, experienced radiologists know what real trouble looks like on a mammogram and how to find it, particularly if other methods have already indicated that trouble exists. All judgments and panic attacks have to be delayed, however, until the pathologist—the doctor who examines under the microscope the actual tissue taken from the lumpectomy—is able to determine what is actually going on. The only good thing about a mammogram is that it locates a problem exactly so that it can be removed without too much damage to the surrounding tissue.

In order to be able to evaluate the usefulness of diagnostic imaging or any other test in health care, doctors look at the percentage of incidence of false positives (i.e., the test is positive but there is no problem) and false negatives (i.e., the test is negative but in fact there is a problem). Mammograms do not look good from this point of view. Eighty percent of women over the age of forty who have mammograms taken end up having biopsies because the radiologist suspects a tumor. The pathologist, however, declares that there is no problem. Whew! All is well: that was a false positive! However, the women to whom this happens end up with a scar on their breasts and they have been thoroughly frightened.

What is even worse, forty percent of mammograms result in false negatives. That is a nightmare: there is a cancer but it is not recognized! The situation is even more dangerous for women with dense breast tissue due to extensive fibroids. There is an eighty percent chance of false negatives for them: their dense fibroid tissue is hiding the tumor.

In light of this we can understand why doctors insist on annual mammograms. They think that the risk of breast cancer is considerable, and they know that their imaging method is not very good. A mammogram is an X-ray image, an image of very complex shadows that vary in density and shape. It takes a long time to learn how to read these X-rays well, and it is a tiring occupation.[6] Borderline cases become judgment calls, and an error would endanger a woman's life. That is why reasonable radiologists recommend biopsies so frequently.

Thermograms, on the other hand, have only a nine percent chance of false negatives or false positives. This is due to the fact that thermograms are objective, exact scientific measurements of heat. The temperatures of both breasts undergo a computerized analysis. All temperature variations within one breast are compared up to a tenth of a degree to the temperature variations within the breast on the contralateral side, even if the autonomic challenge is not positive. As the patient returns for regular check-ups, the measurements from the preceding thermograms are always compared to the current ones via the same detailed analysis.

Thermography not only reveals the presence of cancerous tissue, it gives us two further categories of information. If a thermogram reveals an area of significant heat difference within a breast that turns out to be negative after the autonomic challenge, it still would be considered a problem, but not a dangerous one. This finding could be due to a premenstrual or menopausal hormone imbalance, which would be a physiological problem, a problem in how the breast works. This problem would not have caused a change in the actual tissue of the breast yet, and it can be treated successfully. There is no other imaging that can show such a small problem.

The heat difference could also be due to an injury or an infection, which would be an anatomical problem, actual tissue damage that also can be treated. A naturopath would recommend regular monitoring of these kinds of problems at least three or four times a year.

We can conclude from this that if a thermogram showed a negative autonomic challenge but in fact a cancer was developing (a false negative), the woman would be taking another thermogram in three or four months, as her breasts are being monitored. The naturopath would examine the exact same hot area that he identified in the preceding thermogram and, of course, would perform another autonomic challenge, thus reducing the chances of another false negative. This is only true, though, if the patient returns for regular tests, which I highly recommend.

If the naturopath found a thermogram with a positive autonomic challenge, he or she would refer the patient for an ultrasound, which would confirm if the area of concern was indeed a solid tumor or just a fluid-filled cyst. If the ultrasound showed a fluid-filled cyst we would know that the thermogram had given us a false positive. This would not stop the doctor from continuing to monitor the breast because there was a heat difference. If the ultrasound showed a solid tumor, a mammogram would locate it exactly and a lumpectomy would be performed to find out what is truly happening.

A cancer that is diagnosed that way will most probably be very small and curable by lumpectomy. I need to repeat again that only a pathologist who looks at actual breast cells can tell with almost one hundred percent certainty if a cancer is present or not. I say "almost" because human error exists. The chance for the occurrence of human error can be reduced by having the lumpectomy tissue divided into two or three parts and sent to two or three different pathology labs. I would also insist that two or three pathologists evaluate the same tissue. That's the course of action that I would choose for myself, and I recommend it to my patients.

fibroid tumors of the uterus and their consequences

FIBROID TUMORS OF the uterus are thought to be a consequence of a hormonal imbalance similar to the imbalances already mentioned: too much estrogen, not enough progesterone. Fibroids can develop surreptitiously in the pre-menopausal and peri-menopausal years; they can start developing as early as the late thirties or early forties if there is a serious hormone imbalance. They can be palpated during a good pelvic exam, even if they are small. Fibroids are not supposed to be a problem if they remain small. Often gynecologists do not even mention when they find small ones. There could be one, there could be many. They could be attached to the outside wall of the uterus, they could be attached to the inner wall of the uterus, they could be located within the muscular wall of the uterus. Fibroids become problematic when they enlarge or multiply, which they will do if the hormone imbalance persists and/or worsens. In some cases they can grow up to the size of a large grapefruit and more; in others they can remain small but proliferate and invade the uterine walls, making pregnancy difficult or impossible. A Rolfer or an osteopath or anybody skilled in really looking at a body can literally see them, if the fibroids are large enough. One might think: The lady looks okay, but the abdomen is not really fitting the picture. It sticks out a little too much, even though there is good muscle tone; the abdomen bulges low. If the fibroids are located anteriorly or laterally they can be palpated from the superficial abdominal wall because they are dense and feel hard.

Fibroids do not cause symptoms in the early stages. If women are told by their gynecologists that fibroids are present, they are usually also told that the problem "will go away" soon after menopause starts. This is true . . . unless the hormone imbalance worsens and the fibroids become too large too quickly, cause pain, and interfere with the other pelvic organs, in which case they will need to be removed surgically. Often the latter part of this sentence is not even mentioned in the preliminary diagnosis. If things evolve very unfavorably the entire uterus might need to be removed, which would leave a woman maimed, in my humble opinion, and unbalanced and prolapsed in all her remaining pelvic and abdominal organs. That is my opinion. I must say, though, that a hysterectomy can be a godsend to a woman who needed to free herself from the compression on her other organs caused by a heavy fibrosed uterus. In her case any consequent imbalances can be treated. I would certainly only choose surgery for myself—and advise it for my patients—if it really was the only choice possible.

A good reason to find out about small uterine fibroids and treat them with bio-identical hormones to stop their growth is that they will leave the uterus not only large and heavy but also uneven. A shifted uterus will affect the position of the sacrum via the utero-sacral ligaments and, eventually, may cause pain in the low back and the sacro-iliac joints. Even if the fibroid is not unevenly located, it will increase the weight of the uterus and will cause abnormal front-to-back weight-bearing and soft tissue strain, which can cause the uterus and the adjacent organs to prolapse, to sag. This can cause crowding and problems in the joints of the hips, the sacrum, and the lumbar spine. I have already described these relationships in the previous chapter about pain during menstruation. Allow me to insist and elaborate: the malposition of the sacro-iliac joints caused by the uneven pull of a fibroid will recur monthly in a menstruating woman and will gradually become chronic in a post-menopausal woman if the fibroid is large enough. A skilled practitioner can correct the imbalances of the bones and joints and the position of the uterus through rebalancing the utero-sacral ligaments. If the unevenly weighted uterus remains unchanged, however, the imbalance of the sacrum will return again and again and eventually become permanent. It will affect not only the sacro-iliac joints but also the entire pelvic area and the legs. A consequent contraction of the piriformis muscles can exert pressure on either sciatic nerve and can cause sciatica, a nasty acute pain from the buttocks to the knee and sometimes even to the foot.

Doctors would rarely conclude that a case of sciatica is due to an unevenly positioned uterus or a moderate uterine fibroid. In fact, all kinds of positions of the uterus are considered "within normal limits" by gynecologists because the uterus can function normally in various positions. Western medicine is practiced according to systems, and everybody knows that the reproductive system has no bearing on the musculoskeletal system, right? We can spin this tale even further: sciatic pain in one leg will make a person favor the painful leg by carrying more weight on the pain-free leg, causing the hip bones to become uneven; and this predisposes the woman to coxoarthrosis, arthritis of the hip. This can also affect the ligaments that attach the hips to the lower lumbar vertebrae, and trouble can wander up the back.

Let's also have a closer look at how a fibrosed uterus can affect the adjacent organs. An enlarged, hard, and heavy uterus can put pressure on the bladder and even crowd it, causing the woman to feel the need to urinate frequently. It may also interfere with normal voiding of the rectum by masking "the call of nature," the normal sensation of pressure indicating the need to defecate. A consequently overfilled rectum would really not help the situation at all. Saddest of all, this may make intercourse very uncomfortable. One would then literally be between a rock and a hard place, right?

Two potentially serious problems relating to fibroid tumors need to be mentioned: abnormal bleeding and misdiagnosis. Abnormal bleeding always causes trouble, the least of which is anemia, with accompanying serious fatigue. The worst possible scenario with abnormal bleeding would be that the fibroid is really a cancerous tumor of the uterus. If a fibroid exists it needs to be evaluated carefully via a pelvic exam and diagnostic imaging, mostly MRI and ultrasound. Diagnostic imaging should never be considered too expensive by any responsible doctor. It shows us the reality of the situation.

The second serious problem related to fibroid tumors is that even the best palpation may not lead to an accurate diagnosis. The pelvic organs are very close to each other and one might want to think one has found a fibroid, because it is not a serious problem. There may instead be a small tumor on a neighboring organ. The diagnostic images would simply reveal this.

I asked my gynecologist why she chose gynecology. She said: because regular gynecological exams give women a chance to survive serious problems. So, next time you go for your yearly Pap test, ask about the specific position of your uterus. Is it rotated? Is it prolapsed? Is it bent or turned sideways? Ask about the presence of fibroids, even very small ones. And remember, as with other problems caused initially by hormone imbalance, fibroid tumors will continue to grow if the hormone imbalance is not corrected. After a fibroid has been removed a new fibroid tumor may reappear if the hormone imbalance is not corrected. A small fibroid can disappear if hormone balance is restored.[7]

I have a patient who walks around with a large fibroid. It really feels like she has a large hard orange in her belly. She has serious back pain almost all the time. I can make her feel better for a few days by normalizing the sacrum and the spine. She is still too scared to have the fibroid removed. I am encouraging her to do it. She was considering it and she was getting second opinions about how to proceed when a gynecologist declared that the removal of the fibroid would have no impact on her back pain. Can you see that this gynecologist is dead wrong? Not only that, with just one sentence she obliterated my careful encouragement toward surgery! I have to start from scratch! The patient needs to understand her options: living with recurring and serious back pain that will compromise her mobility and most probably damage her back and her hip joints with time, or submitting herself to surgery with its inherent risks.

the trouble with the "flatlanders"

The charm of knowledge would be small if so much
shame did not have to be overcome on the road to it.
—FRIEDRICH NIETZSCHE

ASKING YOUR GYNECOLOGIST about the specific and detailed position and characteristics of your uterus during your annual pelvic exam could either bother or intrigue her or him. If your doctor is part of a harassed practice where women's annual exams are just routine, he or she might barely be able to suppress a snicker. You might be asked why on Earth you could possibly be interested in a thing like that.

There was a time when humans believed that the Earth was a flat surface, and that chaos lurked beyond the oceans at the edges of the world. Nobody knew where it was exactly, but monsters had been seen and the ships that apparently ventured too close were never seen again. They were supposed to have fallen over the edge into chaos.

In the Renaissance, scientists of different cultures and religions had more contact with each other, and the Catholic church in Europe lost its dominion over scientific thinking. As a result, scientific thinking took great strides, and the Earth was perceived as a sphere and as part of a large universe. The flat-Earth myth went underground. It was also still possible then for one brilliant person to know all that could be known.

Nowadays we have arrived at a level where many of us are, again, baffled by the nature of reality. The edges of the macro- and the micro-cosmos are threatening to touch the absurd. The different fields of science have become so extensive that it is not possible by any stretch of the imagination to know everything. A dialogue between two scientists, specialists in one field, may seem poetry at best to an eavesdropping third scientist from a totally different field. This is true for our work too. Ancient and modern medicine and all the specialties, subspecialties, and related fields have become more and more specialized and compartmentalized. It is increasingly rare in the Western world to find an MD who likes to practice "general medicine," who wants to be the "house doctor" or the "family doctor." This part of medicine seems to slowly be slipping toward naturopathy, homeopathy, acupuncture, Ayurvedic medicine, or herbalism, at least for the educated middle class. But as soon as there is true organ damage, or as soon as there is a life-threatening condition, the doctor who knows us as a person refers us to a specialist, and he or she often recedes into the background because there is very little dialogue between specialists and other practitioners. Within the actual field of modern medicine, there is sometimes very good dialogue. More often, instead of dialogue, there is division of competency. Let's look at a few examples: The dentist refers to the orthodontist or to the oral surgeon, the gynecologist refers to the breast specialist, the physiatrist refers to the neurologist who refers to the neurosurgeon or the orthopedic surgeon, the internist refers to the cardiologist or to the proctologist, etc.

When people get older they often have several doctors taking care of their organ problems. Nobody, however, really takes care of the whole patient and oversees her health, unless the patient is either lucky or rich and can afford to see a doctor just to speak

about her options. Often nobody notices that medications prescribed by different doctors have interactive or cumulative side
effects. Nobody notices that the patient may have left out major
parts of the medical history when speaking to a specialist . . . and
it happens that people simply die of the consequences of very
good medical decisions that damage related organs or exhaust
the patient's vitality. Are such disasters necessarily inevitable?

The chances of people staying healthy longer and having good
vitality rise with regular checkups with practitioners like the so-
called "alternative" doctors (acupuncturists, homeopaths, etc.)
who are not trained to take care of life-threatening emergencies
but who are definitely trained to take care of functional trouble
and are well positioned to notice an ominous change. If they
are worth their salt they will also know the reputable medical
specialists in case a referral is needed. These practitioners also
know how to re-equilibrate the body after emergencies have
been treated. This is still very controversial, and here is where
"flatlander" thinking rears its ugly head from the edge of chaos.

I will not speak badly about modern Western medicine *per se*.
Far from it! Just consider the newest developments, like Magnetic
Resonant Imaging, endoscopic surgery, embryonic cell research,
and traumatology, just to mention a few. Should I, God forbid,
break a leg, I would not go first to my acupuncturist, no matter
how much I love and respect her. But I would see her as soon as
the plaster dried to be treated for the shock to my system.

What I want to point out is the lack of inter-specialty com-
munication and the lack of respect. An MD may think that
chiropractic, acupuncture, or Rolfing are nothing but hogwash,
because whatever ails the patient has not developed enough yet to
actually cause tissue damage. "Oh, I see, you are treating people
for problems that they don't have yet. That's very good for business!" This thinking is unfortunate and exists only because many
Western medical doctors still know mostly nothing of substance

about the modern alternative medical practices that originate in Taoist and Ayurvedic philosophy (from the Greek *philo,* meaning "love," and *sophia,* meaning "wisdom"), in shamanism, and in herbalism. These schools of thought represent more than three millennia of collective thinking and clinical experience. Grumpy conventional doctors might ascribe any healing coming from those fields to "mere spontaneous remission" (and since when is spontaneous remission low-class healing?). But they are not alone! Osteopaths may think poorly of chiropractors and vice versa, and physical therapists may warn people against Rolfing. Is such prejudice really due to ignorance, or is it pigheadedness, or are those the same?

Let's look at an example of how these attitudes can jeopardize patients' health. One day, a sweet little old lady in her eighties whom I had treated off and on for joint pain and stiffness for several years showed up demanding that I open a window, saying that my room was really hot. That was not normal for her: usually she felt very cold and rushed to get under the heated flannel sheet on the treatment table. On this day she was flushed. That also was not normal for her: usually she was pale. I asked if she felt okay. She said she didn't but couldn't tell me anything about it. I took her pulse, which usually was a little fast and slight. That day it was very strong and definitely faster. I asked about her normal blood pressure. She told me that it had been on the low side for years. I took her blood pressure and it was far from the low side. I told her that she needed to call her doctor that day, and that she should ask to be referred to the cardiologist for a checkup. During our treatment session, I treated her gingerly, making sure that I did not do anything to raise her pulse. I called her the next day to make sure she had an appointment to see her doctor.

When she came back two weeks later, she told me that her doctor had said that she did not need to see the cardiologist and that, for her age, her condition was normal. I asked if she had insisted that her condition was not normal, that usually she had low blood pressure and that this was a rather recent change. She said that she did insist and she did say that her chiropractor sent her. She added that in the course of the slightly heated interaction she was asked how long she wanted to live anyway. She said that she had answered, "Long enough to survive you!" and left slamming the door. I said, "Good girl!"

I decided to call my osteopath, describe the situation, and ask her to examine my patient. I also asked if I could observe their consultation myself, so I could see how my colleague handled the situation. During our session, the osteopath definitely agreed that the lady should not just sit by with such a high blood pressure and, in front of us, got on the phone, blasted her way through secretarial stalling, and gave her piece of mind rather coldly to the doctor in question. Things worked out for the patient, she took blood pressure medication, and she died, many years later, of an unrelated problem.

All fields of true knowledge have become very vast, but the chaos at the edges, believe me, is becoming less and less threatening. The edge of somebody's knowledge has a good chance of touching the edge of somebody else's knowledge. We alternative practitioners can all contribute to reducing the risks of "flatlandering" by talking to each other. We might be surprised to see how curious other practitioners and doctors are about us and our work. Some medical doctors know perfectly well that they have replaced the patient with the organ. They know that what practitioners of manipulative medicine do with their hands can be totally complementary to many problems at hand, pun intended.

When I was in chiropractic college we ran out of X-ray films to study for the chiropractic boards. We knew all the X-rays we had in our own library by heart: we could call out the diagnosis after seeing the image for half a second. We needed X-rays we had never seen. Someone had the great idea to just boldly prance into the San Francisco Medical School Radiology Department, pretending that we were medical students. Once we got there, the four or five of us took the spinal and the pelvic X-rays, read them, and discussed things with more and more enthusiasm until we ended up forgetting where we were. The medical students started to eavesdrop on us and finally asked: "Who are you guys?" Busted! We thought we would be escorted to the door. But no: they really wanted to know why such detailed analysis of relationship between the different parts of the body was so important to us. We told them. One of them started by first checking his surroundings carefully and then he came closer and whispered, "I have had this pain in my back for so long. Do you guys think you could do something about it?"

During one of my annual exams my gynecologist wondered why I needed to know the exact position of my uterus. I told her that I was interested in the position of my uterus precisely because my left sacro-iliac joint had the pesky habit of going out of alignment, and adjustments made to it did not hold very well. I wondered if maybe my uterus was a little crooked and thus pulled on the sacrum via the cervico-sacral ligaments. She said, "Oooh! Well...Yes, your cervix looks just a little turned to the right."

I asked, "Are you willing to rebalance my uterus, if I talk you through it?"

She was. As a gynecologist she was, of course, totally comfortable holding the uterus to evaluate it, to feel the density of its walls, etc. She had, however, never attempted to change the position of a uterus by very lightly pulling on the utero-sacral ligaments. She was surprised and pleased to feel the right cervico-sacral ligament release and so was I, and my sacro-iliac joint held its subsequent adjustment.

Many kinds of variations from normal anatomy are known, of course. Some people have missing or additional vertebrae, some have only one kidney, some have what is called "situs inversus" (that is, their heart is on the right side), some men have only one testicle, some women have a double uterus (try to have a baby with that thing!). People may never be told about minor abnormalities because they do not really matter if they do not cause trouble. Extreme positions of the uterus can fall into the category of abnormalities that cause trouble. You might have a very innocent-looking, slightly crooked uterus, but if it is accompanied by monthly or constant back pain, it is a problem, even if another patient with the same slight imbalance does not have back pain.

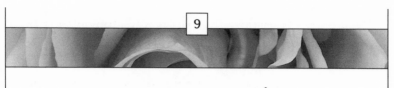

osteoporosis

It is the theory that makes you perceive.
—ALBERT EINSTEIN (1897–1955)

THE OFFICIAL THEORY about osteoporosis is that it is here to stay, that it is a demineralization of bones that commonly happens to many types of post-menopausal women: white, blond, of northern European origin, of slight stature, underweight, living in industrialized countries, sedentary, consuming alcohol, smoking tobacco, etc. Most of this has become common knowledge. One clearly stated risk factor for osteoporosis is being a woman. It just rubs me the wrong way to have to hear that being a woman is a risky thing!

I have not found a convincing explanation yet as to why osteoporosis should happen mostly to post-menopausal women, even though this is commonly observed. I wonder if the observation only began to be made after people had created the theory. Maybe after the theory was in place they started to ignore other pretty good possible causes. Personally I am not certain that osteoporosis is related to menopause. I know young and menstruating women who have poor bone mineralization. The belief that menopause somehow causes osteoporosis could be based on the frequent coincidental occurrence. Osteoporosis could be related to aging, a sedentary lifestyle, and poor nutrition. It does happen to men, but less frequently, and it is mostly seen in men who are sedentary, very old, malnourished, or ill.

What we know specifically is that there are gradually more cells that get rid of old bone (osteoclasts) than cells that create new bone (osteoblasts), which results in a deficient turnover of bone. This condition is attributed to estrogen deficiency but also to calcium and other related mineral deficiencies, to vitamin D deficiency, to poor calcium/magnesium balance, and to lack of weight-bearing exercise. Another theory attributes bone demineralization to a combination of dehydration and excessive consumption of carbonated drinks and acidic foods. In my opinion, strong evidence that osteoporosis is due only to estrogen deficiency is not really established.

Bones are our only solid structural elements; they are the spacers of our muscle tissue; they offer attachment sites for the ligaments and tendons; and they allow us to move around in Earth's gravity field without collapsing. I think that the strength of bones depends equally on adequate nutrition, normal physiology, and the pressure of gravity on our bodies. We have come to understand that weight-bearing physical activity is important to maintain good bone density during our entire lifetime. Bones and gravity are an item, so to speak. Our bones enable us to move in the field of gravity, and we lose them if we are not influenced sufficiently by gravity.

Let's use an extreme example to illustrate the concept. It's not only the lazy, the sick, the sedentary, and the elderly who lose bone mass. Some of our best-trained military people were exposed to osteoporosis: astronauts! As soon as astronauts were cooped up in their capsules and out there away from the Earth's gravitational field, floating around weightlessly, their bodies started a slow process of excreting small amounts of bone-building minerals into their urine. In the course of one lengthy mission a Soviet astronaut lost enough bone tissue to have his ribcage fatally crushed by the pressure of gravity as he re-entered the Earth's gravitational field. Exercise machines have since been designed and added into the space ships to provide our courageous space travelers with weight-bearing exercise to keep their bones sound. So the body seems to know when bones are needed: No gravity? No bones needed! Isn't that something! Who tells our body that it can return to being a cushy mollusk when there is no gravity? Is this caused by the old demon, intelligent design?

The hip joint is a large, strong joint with a very wide range of motion in a healthy person. It is often damaged when people have osteoporosis. Any joint is more likely to be damaged than a straight bone, if we don't respect its design and function. This is true for us all, even for the strongest men. Let's consider the case of a very wild, fun, and macho friend of mine from Europe who let himself get tempted to enjoy cocaine. He liked it so much that he let himself be tempted to sell it to his friends. This being a major illegal activity, he took on the name "Dr. White": his customers would call him under that name to find out when the "medicine" had arrived. About twenty years after we first met I saw Dr. White again; he was in his early fifties. By then he really looked the part. His hair was all white. There was, however, something preternaturally aged in his walk. I inquired about an injury. He said no, he wasn't actually injured. He had had "aseptic necrosis" of both hip joints and they needed to be surgically replaced. This means that the small arteries that fed his hip joints had gradually been so damaged by his destructive habit that they simply degenerated, ceased to exist, and left the bone to become osteoporotic, to disintegrate and collapse. Luckily, he was diagnosed and treated. He had bilateral hip replacement surgery. Also, luckily, he re-learned to enjoy breakfast, lunch, and dinner and he gave up his evening job.

I would like us all to understand that osteoporosis results from nutritional deficiency, physiological malfunctions (which could include hormone deficiency), and "gravitational" deficiency. Any of these will eventually creep up on us if we neglect our need to live intelligently in this well-designed and sensitive body.

the dreaded hip fracture

A COMMON FRACTURE rightfully feared in the presence of osteoporosis is the hip fracture. The "hip fracture" of elderly women is not really a hip fracture at all. It is a fracture of the neck of the femur, the upper end of the thighbone, right where the leg fits into the hip.

This fracture can happen with a fall or any accident in the presence of osteoporosis. Often the fracture actually does not happen because the woman falls; she falls because the bone breaks as she is walking. In this case the neck of the femur is so weak and depleted, it simply cannot bear the impact of one more normal step or of a minor trip. It is clear that such a fracture can only happen to a person who has been developing osteoporosis for a long period of time. There is good reason to fear such a fracture; it is often the last thing that happens to an old lady. After the fracture the patient is unable to move for a long time, and the immobility compromises her general blood circulation. Hospitalized and medicated with mind-numbing pain pills, she might become depressed, she might decline physical therapy, and she might never recover. Anything could kill her at that point—embolism, pneumonia. . . . Twenty percent of all women who suffer a "hip fracture" die within a year, just because they lose their mobility, which always brings about a cascade of trouble for the elderly.

Why is that part of the femur so prone to breaking? In a healthy body it is very sturdy and is supported by extensive ligaments; it is designed to absorb most of the impact of walking, jumping, and running. If people become sedentary for a long time, the joint remains still, and less motion brings about less circulation. This area, being very small, also has very small arteries. The branches of the medial circumflex artery that feed the head and the neck of the femur are quite narrow. Hence the importance of staying mobile and, even more crucial, of doing something that involves moderate effort in order to stimulate the heart and the circulation. Just walking the dog may not be enough. Walking uphill with a little speed would be better. Wearing a backpack with a gradually increasing amount of books would also help. But just walking uses such a small range of the hip joint. Why don't we all find a teacher with a good reputation whom we will see now and then or often so we can learn how to remain really mobile? Many bright people with the well-being of the body in mind have been teaching the restorative aspects of techniques like Tai Chi or Yoga for thousands of years. These and contemporary Western approaches to this noble knowledge—like the Alexander and Feldenkrais techniques, Pilates, and Gyrotonic training—actively engage your mind! You will feel goofy in the beginning and keel out of your alignment if you do not concentrate fully. But you will rediscover the basic design of your physical self and you will enjoy the accelerated circulation. This is not gerbil-like, Sisyphean treadmill-scurrying, not silly busy work that will bore you to tears! With diligence and after some time, when you have become a little more confident, you will gradually see that you are re-creating a mobility that you have not had for a long time, maybe even since you were a child. This would be the case for anybody—young, elderly, sedentary—who is changing his or her ways. One of my elderly Italian colleagues from Venice started his training in Yoga after he was forty years old. The last time I saw him he could stand on his hands and talk to me. When we went for a walk, younger women turned their heads when he sailed by.

A word of caution: Any method that has the power to change the body for the better can also cause injury if it is not done correctly. That means beginning students need teachers. You cannot start training by yourself or by watching a lesson on television or on a DVD if you are just restarting to become more mobile! You need to take a class, and if the lessons cause pain, you need personal attention. It is well worth it to start on a good foot! If mild discomfort is caused, the activity should be reduced and you might use anti-inflammatory herbs as you gradually increase your range. But do not ever give up your mobility! Don't do it, hell no! There is no way back from there!

I learned this lesson in a memorable way from a remarkable patient. I was in my last year as a chiropractic intern, and a friend of mine who had just graduated gave a patient file to me. He said, "This is my bye-bye present to you, Georgette. I am not going to tell you anything about the case. Just remember, it's a present."

I studied the X-rays. The patient was in her eighties. The X-rays showed severe end-stage arthritis in the neck. It looked like the patient had no neck motion left. When the patient came for treatment I walked into the waiting room, expecting to meet a little old lady, bent over, able to look around and orient herself only by turning with her entire torso. I called her name. A blue-eyed lady with wrinkles wearing a blue dress that matched her eyes got up with ease and walked towards me looking right and left quite normally. I muttered, "Oh, I have the wrong X-rays."

She said, "No, you don't." I must have looked baffled. She added, "There's something you don't know," with a cute, smart-ass smile. I was glad to see that she had a sense of humor, because I was not feeling that sharp right then. Inside the treatment room she said that she was a retired physical therapist and that she knew with certainty that if you stop moving an arthritic joint it will degenerate all the way to ankylosis (fusion of the bones in a joint). She showed me the exercises she did every day of her life, without exception. This did not explain the mistake I made when I read the X-ray. There really was no joint space to be seen in any of her neck joints on the X-ray. But when I examined her neck I could feel that there was moderate mobility in all the joints that looked closed on the X-ray. My mistake was that I trusted the X-ray, an image taken during a fraction of a second, and I drew conclusions about reality from that. An X-ray is such an impressive thing, right? It made me mistake the map for the territory. The joint spaces of an old person with arthritis are uneven; there are little hills and outgrowths on the surfaces of the ends of the bones that form the joint. Straight X-ray beams cannot go around these small obstacles, and thus the joints look occluded. If the radiologist had turned the patient this way and that and had taken many views, I might have seen that there were open joint spaces in her neck. However, after what I told you about ionizing radiation, you would understand that nobody in his or her right mind would take multiple X-ray views just to demonstrate the presence of joint spaces.

let's bring nutrition to the foreground

Since osteoporosis, once present, puts the patient at a high risk for fractures, we need to prevent osteoporosis from happening. As we age we need to take vitamin and mineral supplements, and to practice regular weight-bearing activity, of course. Calcium and magnesium are known to be among the most important minerals in bone. The correct amount and balance of these minerals is still being debated and may not matter that much. Other minerals and trace minerals—like strontium, for example—also seem to play an important role. Eating nutritious food, taking supplements, and staying active is sound advice for anybody, women and men; the combination usually works, but not always.

What good is good nutrition if the stomach does not produce enough acids to even start digesting nutrients adequately, be they food or vitamins (which, in fact, are mostly just very concentrated food)? This common condition is known as "achlorhydria." In achlorhydria, the stomach does not produce enough chlorhydric acid, and, just to complicate matters, the condition simply feels like an "acid stomach." Its sufferers buy acid-reducing over-the-counter medication that, of course, makes things even worse. A simple test at the doctor's can reveal the truth about this condition.

And what if, instead, there are simply not enough digestive enzymes to digest the food or the supplements that contain the vitamins and minerals? Your doctor can also test for this, and digestive enzymes can be taken as supplements. The above became most obvious to me when I read the X-ray film of the large intestine of an elderly patient and saw entire undigested vitamin pills still in recognizable shape.

My nutrition teacher in chiropractic college set me on one further interesting route in the search for causes of osteoporosis. Complete proteins are called complete because they contain all the essential amino acids needed to create the cells of the body. All body tissue cells die and are recreated constantly: this is what maintains our physical integrity. Some nutritionists and ortho-molecular physicians think that osteoporosis is a nutritional imbalance related to the metabolism of excessive amounts of complete proteins and the lack of sufficient available calcium. They may have a point, since osteoporosis indeed occurs more frequently among the people who live in the "Western" world, where food, particularly meat, is plentiful.

Complete proteins are found in meat and fish, of course, and in animal products like milk and cheese and eggs. Vegans rely on a clever combination of vegetables, rice, and legumes to provide all the essential amino acids. Vegans also need to take B-12 supplements, since B-12, an essential vitamin for the maintenance of brain and nervous system cells, only exists in animal products. An average-sized person needs more or less forty to sixty grams of pure protein a day for normal mainte-nance. A hard-working or very physically active person will need more protein than a less active person.

An important thing to know is that proteins, unlike fats, are not stored in our bodies. They are construction material that is eliminated as soon as there is no need for it. Excess protein is transformed into urea and excreted in urine. Here comes the link to osteoporosis: We need calcium to make urea. If there is an excess of protein and not enough available loose calcium, the calcium of your bones will be used to make urea. So do white, sedentary, thin, old, and rich ladies literally "piss away" (poetic license) their bones if they eat lots of meat?

An example supporting this train of thought is the fact that Central American Mayan peasant women are said to rarely have osteoporosis. They are very poor and only eat meat on feast days. They mostly eat *frijoles y arroz*, beans and rice, their staples, which eaten together provide complete proteins. They also grow their own vegetables. They do hard physical labor. Anyone who has been to mountainous rural Guatemala will have seen small groups of sturdy women of all ages, walking up and down their steep paths, carrying heavy stuff—vegetables to sell at the market, fabric they made, or whatever—on their backs. On the other hand, Inuit women have a high incidence of osteoporosis. Their staples are fish, right? They also spend much of their time indoors because their world is frozen over during the long Arctic winter months; I am sure their green vegetable growing season is not very long. Or do they simply suffer from malnutrition, considering that the twentieth and twenty-first centuries and the accompanying junk food fashion has arrived there and has largely spared rural Guatemala?

It is good to be reminded that a varied diet containing reasonable amounts of sustainably or organically produced vegetables, fruits, nuts, fermented milk products, few or no refined starches, and not too much natural honey and sugar (as in dehydrated cane juice or grape juice), accompanied by supplements like vitamins, essential fatty acids, and minerals, will nourish you adequately. I must insist on organically or sustainably produced meats. I will not go into the commercial practices of animal husbandry. Suffice to say that I find them appalling and inhumane. Fish should be eaten wild. Don't go near farmed fish and farmed seafood: they are very polluted. There is a small and growing group of people who have started to develop sustainable farming of fish and seafood. Let's wish them luck! Add a little wine and such—just for fun, not too much— then plenty of clean and filtered water and you will thrive.

I am not so sure about cow's milk; it seems to have become "public enemy number one" lately. I agree that commercially produced milk is highly objectionable because, if it does not contain synthetic hormones, it definitely will contain remnants of fertilizers, pesticides, and herbicides from the food the cows ate. Drink milk from cows that are fed organic food, if you like to drink milk. The descendants of people from Northern and Central Europe and other tribes who have raised cattle for centuries and have consumed their milk seem to do well with it. The descendants of people who did not consume milk are often lactose-intolerant, and since many of us don't know all of our racial ingredients anymore, we should proceed with caution. Lactose intolerance causes digestive trouble like bloating, pain, diarrhea, and worse.

Yogurt and other milk products fermented with live bacteria provide good calcium and they also support the healthy bacterial environment of the intestines. These dairy products may still contain lactose, though, unless the fermentation process has lasted longer than forty-eight hours. Commercially produced yogurt may also contain sugar, starch, and stabilizers, which you certainly do not need. Consider making your own organic cow or goat yogurt and letting it ferment for a sufficiently long time, which is two or three days. It is easy to do and the yogurt is delicious.

Many people, even if they are not lactose-intolerant, do not do well with milk, period. This is true even if the milk is very good. The purists among the naturopaths say that milk is very good food for calves, but not for humans; that it actually is a foreign substance to humans, an allergen, and that it affects our immune system adversely. They say that recurrent infant ear infections, for example, are caused by milk consumption.

Entire civilizations do not have or use milk, other than mother's milk, of course. They get their calcium from vegetables. The calcium content of green vegetables is higher per weight than the calcium content of milk, and it is more bio-available, i.e., easy to digest and assimilate.

Another substance that is a constant preoccupation for nutrition experts is sugar. Humans do like sweet things. This is because the first food we know, mother's milk (or its replacement), is sweet, nutritious, and easy to assimilate. I will speak more about the digestion of sugar, so for the moment let's briefly look at its assimilation: Simple sugar, glucose, is the fuel for our brain. So why, oh why, are nutritionists so uptight about it? Because refined sugar as we know it—the stuff we use to sweeten our food—is not really a food that our body knows; it has only been available since people learned to extract it from the complete food—sugar cane, beets, corn, or other plants that also contain fiber, vitamins, and minerals. Sugar that does not come from bees was first heard of in Persia in the sixth century, and mass production only started in the fifteenth century in the Caribbean. Before that sweeteners were honey and dried fruit or other plants, which are complex substances.

The sugars we use now are very simple molecules that can enter our bloodstream rapidly and in large quantities—and that is why they cause trouble. When sugar (let's say only a teaspoon of it) enters our bloodstream via the capillaries of the digestive system, only a very small amount of it, less than one percent, is used and metabolized to give you an energy lift. This is the well-known, short-lived "sugar high." Not a big deal, no problem for the young and sturdy. Some of us like these sugar highs. We enhance the sugar high with a little coffee boost to the adrenal glands, which accelerates the heart. How exciting! Caffeinated soft drinks, same combo, have become the staple of well-functioning businesses and are consumed massively by children and adolescents.

The leftover ninety-nine percent of our teaspoon of sugar invariably creates a small emergency situation in the body. The presence of high sugar in the bloodstream triggers a quick release of insulin from the pancreas. Insulin and sugar are made into fat and stored away. When this emergency procedure is repeated too often and the response begins to slow down, people are left with high blood sugar and they eventually develop diabetes. It probably takes a genetic predisposition for this to happen. But it happens as people grow older, and it happens to more of us today because we consume increasingly more sugar. We also see far more young children who are overweight and diabetic.

From a nutritional point of view, refined sugar is not food; it's just a pointless emergency. Yes, the fat that was sent to storage could be used later. It is, however, hard to reach that fat—real hunger and real sweat are needed to get to the storage. Mostly fat just hangs out and grows. Many people become heavy very gradually... it is normal to become a little pudgy as time goes by, right? Obesity with all its destructive consequences is not that far from here.

I want to invite all of us to really get to know the basics. Observe your established eating habits, looking for ones that may have lost their value. It is easy to isolate them: you simply do not feel so great right after you eat certain foods or a little later. Bust out of the ghetto of prejudice about nutrition! Become creative with food! It can change your life. There is plenty of information available about great nutrition and great cooking. I personally admire, applaud, and try to emulate the teachings of the California Nouvelle Cuisine School.[8] These chefs and home cooks insist on the use of organic, local, and sustainably grown food that is in season.

For dessert, I will impart to you the maxim of my most radical nutrition teacher from chiropractic college: "Read the ingredients of all packaged food! If you can't pronounce the words, throw the package away! If you do not know what the words mean, throw the package away! If any ingredient is fructose, maltose, saccharose, lactose—anything ending with 'ose'—throw the package away! Conclusion: If it comes in a package, throw it away!"[9]

dehydration and fluid retention

Water, like air, food, and sleep, is absolutely essential for normal physiology. In the hot Sahara Desert a healthy strong man can die within a day from dehydration. The amount of internal fluid is almost always looked at when health is evaluated. In your lab reports you can see it under the heading "specific gravity."

Most healers I have met recommend drinking at least two liters or two quarts of water a day and specify that more is needed in hot weather or with strenuous effort. When this was told to me I said, "Okay, I'll do that, but I will spend much of my time on the loo!" The answer was, "Yes, but with time your body will adapt and your health will increase." Since that time I have gradually become aware of the fact that lack of water is adverse to my well-being, to my concentration, and to my digestion. Mild dehydration can be the cause of diffuse headaches, minor peripheral swelling, slight muscle pain, constipation, and serious grumpiness.

A foolproof way to tell if your water intake is sufficient is to evaluate the quantity, color, smell, and clarity of your urine and the frequency of your urination. Do you urinate at least six to eight times in a day? Is your urine really transparent and pale yellow? It should have a light smell that dissipates fast from the room. If you really want to know more you could do what the traditional Chinese and Tibetan doctors do. Choose a clear glass jar, urinate inside, close the jar tightly (rather important), and hold it against the light. Evaluate the urine in there. The only color acceptable is pale yellow; it should be transparent with very minor or no floating debris, and no foam that persists for more than half a minute or so after you have shaken it. Your findings can vary as the day goes by: in the morning, just after you get up, the color is always a little more concentrated, but it still should be rather transparent.

Food can have varying effects on this, of course. Red beets will color urine pink and can cause scares about the presence of blood. Asparagus will give it a very strong smell; B vitamins will impart an intense canary-yellow color; medication can alter urine in many ways. All of this should be temporary and should pass, pun intended, within a day after the food has been consumed or the medication is stopped.

Many women choose to not drink, even if they are thirsty, because they want to avoid having to wander off to the loo all the time. How ill advised! Serious chronic dehydration by itself can make body tissues too salty. This condition is not just an accumulation of normal salt but of all kinds of metal salts—like magnesium salts and others—which cause water to accumulate in the dehydrated tissue. The accumulated fluid just stays there. It does not benefit the body at all; it is locked up because of the salt. This is what makes a dehydrated person look "fat." If you palpate tissue full of fluid it feels similar to squeezing a kid's water bomb (balloon tightly filled with water)—the tissue does not have the familiar love-handle squishiness. This state is called edema, a sign of abnormal kidney and liver function that affects the entire physiology including the hormone balance. The vicious cycle becomes apparent, doesn't it?

My mother's friends used to ask their doctors to prescribe them Lasix, a prescription medication that forces fluid out via the kidneys, so they could fit in their elegant evening clothes when they were premenstrual. How dangerous! Diuretic medication changes the filtration rate of your kidneys, opens the floodgates wide, and makes you release all kinds of important substances that you need. Furthermore, avoiding water and/or taking diuretic herbs or medication does not really take care of the causes of fluid retention. It is just one more way to kill the messenger.

Fluid retention can be seen in body parts where fat does not commonly accumulate, like the ankles or the eye sockets. A simple test is very revealing: poke a swollen ankle with your pointed finger for a second or two. Your finger might leave a little pit that lasts for some time. This is called pitting edema. It is due to fluid stagnation. The time it takes for the pit to go away is a common measure of how serious the fluid retention is. There should be zero pitting edema in the legs of a healthy, well-hydrated person.

We have seen that premenstrual fluid retention caused by dehydration and/or hormone imbalance can temporarily make the abdomen, breasts, and legs swell quite noticeably. Peri-menopausal fluid retention is quite different in that it can become persistent and apparently unmanageable, particularly if the woman has decided to use conventional hormone replacement therapy. Some women are still being told that, in spite of the discomfort caused by the hormones, they need to remain on hormone replacement therapy into their old age to prevent the progression of osteoporosis and heart damage.

The practice of treating menopausal symptoms with hormones was first started in the 1950s.[10] It quickly became an established procedure: find out what's missing and supplement with something as identical as possible that has been researched and synthesized by the pharmaceutical industry. This is symptom suppression, a good old-world, Western medicine approach. It worked well on a superficial level. The artificial hormone supplementation created the desired state since the symptoms "went away": end of problem. The actual cause of the problem was not looked for, because the direct symptomatic approach, widely used by most doctors, worked very well. For about thirty years all seemed well, but finally a connection was made between routine hormone supplementation for menopausal problems and the development of breast and uterine cancer. The advantages of hormone replacement therapy that doctors once believed in, like protection from heart disease and memory problems, do not exist.

Menopausal problems are usually caused by severe hormonal imbalance, but they can be the result of many other causes. These could be functional problems of organs such as the liver, the adrenal glands, the thyroid gland, and even the pituitary gland. The complexity of this has become the object of interest of a relatively new school of thinking, the orthomolecular approach. I have mentioned this important point already. Orthomolecular doctors treat with natural, plant-based substances, which could be hormones or food supplements that replace what is missing in the body, if and only if it is missing, and only for as long as it is missing. This is not easy to do. It involves detailed history-taking, expensive lab studies, medication compounded by a pharmacist for an individual patient, regular monitoring, adjustments of dosage, and a supportive diet. It takes time to achieve good results, and the treatment is expensive. It also calls for patient compliance—the patient's willingness to enter into such a relationship with the doctor and to follow directions.

Orthomolecular medicine has been practiced for at least thirty years but remains relatively unknown. Some of my patients in their seventies and eighties still take their Premarin and Provera (synthetic estrogens and progesterone). They will not stop taking their pills because years ago their doctor told them not to. They are afraid of hot flashes and night sweats, and they are convinced that their bones will fall apart as soon as they stop hormone replacement therapy. I had the opportunity to see the result of this gradual transition in friends and relations from other countries as they go through menopause with conventional hormone therapy. Since I do not see them often, their transformation has been shocking. All of them, without exception, gained weight and felt unwell and were nonetheless resigned to taking their pills out of sheer fear that all would become worse if they stopped. On a more somber note: I have had the opportunity to dissect female cadavers. Often the parts that looked from the outside like they were invested with adipose tissue really did not have any fat cells: instead, the tissue was gelatinous and watery.

There has been a great deal of progress in the field of natural or bio-identical hormone replacement therapy and in the field of supplements like vitamins, essential fatty acids, and herbs. Using these tools, acupuncturists, herbalists, homeopaths, Ayurvedic practitioners, and naturopaths with experience can help alleviate problems arising from dehydration and fluid retention.

It is important to consult a practitioner in case of obvious and persistent fluid retention because there are many possible causes for this other than hormone imbalance and/or dehydration. Fluid retention could be caused by poor digestion and/or poor absorption, as well as liver, kidney, or heart damage in varying degrees of seriousness. Fluid retention can also be due to many other diseases, to alcoholism, and to any kind of substance abuse or malnutrition.

a common intestinal malfunction causing fluid retention

We must never forget that what the patient takes beyond his power to digest does harm.
—DR. SAMUEL GEE, 1839–1911

LET'S BE DISTRACTED from problems specific to women by a very common intestinal malabsorption problem that mostly goes unrecognized. It can cause gradual and persistent abdominal fluid retention. It is not related to menopause, but it can become indistinguishable from fluid retention caused by hormone imbalance if it happens simultaneously.

Stay with me, I have to explain this in a rather convoluted way. The problem at hand develops because—for reasons we will see below—the intestine gradually stops completely digesting and absorbing a certain kind of common starch. A starch molecule consists of many glucose molecules linked to each other in various combinations.

Glucose is the sugar that our body uses as fuel, the substance that gives us energy to run the physiology, so to speak. It is the only food that does not need digestion; it is small enough to be absorbed readily as it is. For example, if patients feel major stress before a surgery, it may not only be the fear of the surgery that causes them to tremble and sweat. It may be because they had to fast for up to twelve hours before surgery and hence have the panicky feeling that goes with very low blood sugar. Nurses know this well. They give such patients intravenous glucose, and the strong feeling of panic disappears very quickly, almost as soon as the glucose hits the bloodstream.

One major function of the digestive system is to slice large starch molecules into single glucose molecules and absorb them. There are two main kinds of starches in our diet, amylopectin and amylose. Amylose is very easy to digest. It has a simple, almost linear molecular structure with maybe just a few side arms. It can look like a stick or a tree branch. Contact between amylose and its digestive enzymes is easily established. The starch in most vegetables is amylose. Vegetables are nutritious and contain vitamins and minerals galore. They are digested easily. The undigested remnants of vegetables are eliminated easily because their high fiber content provides bulk, which stimulates the intestinal muscles. The size of vegetables is misleading because they contain a great deal of water, which is good because it hydrates you and bad because you actually eat much less than you think you do and you get hungry more rapidly. Vegetables also spoil quickly because of their unstable structure.

The second kind of starch, amylopectin, is quite different. Amylopectin is the starch that is found in all grains and flours, corn and rice, potatoes and potato-like vegetables such as yams. The molecular structure of this type of starch is complex and very stable; it contains many chains of glucose molecules that have multiple branches and stabilizing links. The molecule of an amylopectin starch looks like a ball of yarn. Its digestion can take a long time.

The characteristics of amylopectin starches have been crucial to the development of human civilization. The gradual coming into existence of agriculture and settlements, then community living with leisure time to self-reflect and come up with decorations and art, is largely due to the fact that humans found a way to grow grains and store them for a long time. Grains and/or their storage containers are found in most archeological digs around the first human settlements. Grains could be dried and taken on migrations to be sown later; new sites could be settled, new towns could be built if good soil was found.

Grains are also very nutritious. Due to their amylopectin content, grains are digested slowly, so that glucose is steadily released into the bloodstream over a long period of time, thus providing many hours of energy. Grains are the ideal food to eat when doing hard, sustained, physical labor.

These wonderful characteristics of the amylopectin starches—dense structure and strong molecular bonds—make them a liability when they enter a digestive system that cannot handle them. In this case these starches remain for many days undigested in the intestine. They do not just linger, they cause trouble.

Undigested and unabsorbed amylopectin starches that linger in the intestines cause abdominal fluid retention and eventually general peripheral swelling. This is accompanied by very noticeable discomforts like abdominal distention, burps, persistent gas, and gas pain, which can start soon after eating and persist for hours. The intestinal transit, which is the extent of time that passes between ingestion and elimination, will gradually lengthen and can end up lasting for two or three days. For some people this deteriorating state of digestion can go on unnoticed for a very long time. Or do people simply refuse to notice that certain everyday foods make them feel unwell and constipate them? If unattended, this problem will gradually degenerate into chronic constipation, alternating eventually with pain and diarrhea. If the situation really worsens, irritable bowel syndrome can develop. At that stage of the problem even simple disaccharides—sugars that are formed of just two molecules, like table sugar, fructose, and lactose—also become quasi-indigestible.

The malabsorption problem I am describing happens most

commonly to elderly people. The patients have very low stomach acids, a deficient enzyme system, or maybe even a slowly developing hypersensitivity to starches. The resulting "burping and farting disease" is no laughing matter. It can end up causing muscle aches and stiff joints, even full-blown arthritis, headaches and fatigue, skin rashes and psoriasis—all the common old-age ailments that one is supposed to put up with, right? A good doctor or a good alternative practitioner can recognize these intestinal toxicity symptoms, perform the appropriate testing, prescribe herbs, enzymes, probiotics, and vitamins, and advise a diet change before the problem becomes a serious pathology.

The reason I bring this up here is that this problem can happen to anybody, even strong young people, for a very specific reason: it can be the delayed consequence of repeated antibiotic treatments for unrelated ailments. It can start months after antibiotic treatment is stopped.

We need a good and useful example. Let's take cystitis, a urinary tract infection, a common reason to take antibiotics for young and sexually active women. Let's see how surreptitiously but inevitably the intestines can get damaged. Women have a short urethra and it is located very close to the anus. This makes it possible for bacteria from the large intestine to accidentally enter the bladder during intercourse. In most cases these bacteria are *Escherichia coli.* (Bacteria sometimes carry the name of the person who discovered them. These are named after Dr. Escherich from Austria.) They live in the colon. So the bacteria's Latin name means: "Escherich's, belonging to the colon," a.k.a. "E. coli" for family and friends.

It is a simple fact that we share our world with bacteria. Our bodies are their natural habitat—we are their planet, so to speak. They mostly don't hurt us if we have an adequate immune system and if they remain in the area where they normally live. *E. coli* are dominant in the colon, *Pneumocystis carinii* live in the lungs, Staphylococcus—even the very dangerous *Staphylococcus aureus*—can live on the skin without causing trouble. These bacteria are called commensals, from the Latin words *cum,* meaning "together" and *mensa,* meaning "table": they literally "eat at the same table." Some of them are part of our daily food. We know about the ones in cheese, like *Penicillium camemberti,* and we know about Acidophilus in yogurt. We sometimes call those bacteria "probiotics," from the Latin root *bio,* meaning "life." *Escherichia coli* are necessary probiotic bacteria for us, because they help with the end stage of digestion.

The probiotic *E. coli* is a benevolent Dr. Jekyll as long as it lives in the large intestine. If it enters into the bladder, it becomes a pathogenic Mr. Hyde. (*Pathos* is a Greek word meaning "suffering," and *genesis* is Greek for "birth or origin"). As a carrier of disease *E. coli* attacks the walls of the bladder and causes urinary tract infections. If it manages to make its way up the ureters into the kidneys, it can cause a life-threatening infection.

If you have a bladder infection, your doctor will first give you a commonly prescribed broad-spectrum antibiotic. Antibiotic and radiation treatment in the medical field can be compared to nuclear bombs in warfare. They are not very specific weapons. They are designed to do a necessary, fast, and dirty job. Broad-spectrum antibiotics aim to eliminate a large variety of bacteria. In the process they create destruction and leave desolation behind them. As soon as it is clear that there is an infection in the body it is common practice to just "nuke" it. Before administering the antibiotics, doctors who are worth their salt will also take a minute sample of the diseased part, a blood sample, or in this case, a sample of urine before prescribing the antibiotic. They will send it to the lab to find out if the antibiotic prescribed is really made for the suspected bacteria because, just judging from the symptoms, they cannot be certain that *E. coli* is causing the problem. This is called a sensitivity test. If there is a serious infection the doctor cannot wait for the lab results, in this case because a urinary tract infection is very painful and would threaten the kidneys if allowed to spread. As soon as the antibiotic enters the bloodstream it takes care of the infection within hours. It will kill off almost all the *E. coli* in the bladder and, of course, also almost all the *E. coli* in the large intestine. It will cause serious havoc among many other bacteria since it addresses a large spectrum of them, and it will kill many beneficial bacteria too.

To make a long story short: in this case the patient has no other choice but to leave the large intestine exposed to malfunction because the *E. coli* must be killed to save the bladder and the kidneys. Those of us who are aware of the problem take massive amounts of Acidophilus and other probiotics once the bladder infection has healed to re-seed the large intestine with favorable bacteria. This does not always work, mostly because we do not know how long we need to supplement ourselves. We also have no way to assess if those probiotics are actually alive when we take them. Eventually we just stop because we are feeling well . . . and the chances are that it is too early to stop.

To really understand antibiotic use for bacterial management, I insist that it be compared and contrasted to nuclear warfare. As I said above, a common antibiotic is never exactly matched solely to the bacteria it is supposed to destroy. It is an indiscriminate weapon and, like a nuclear bomb, it will create massive overkill. Both weapons do destroy the enemy but not only the enemy, by far: they destroy almost everything in the area. You may have seen documentation about Hiroshima and Nagasaki and how these bombs wiped out all structures and all life, human, animal, and plant. The areas hit by these kinds of bombs need an extremely long time to return to their previous states and there are very few survivors. This is where the similarities of both kinds of warfare stop.

Let's contrast the information regarding the aftermaths. In the case of nuclear weapons, the radioactivity seriously damages any survivors' health, down to their ability to reproduce, because of DNA damage. A return to normal physiology became impossible for the heavily irradiated Japanese survivors. They were advised not to attempt to have children after the extent of their injuries was understood.

Antibiotics, on the other hand, do not emit ionizing radiation. Bacteria are very small creatures and, by nature, they have an impressive capacity to constantly mutate their DNA to adapt to circumstances. Bacteria were on Earth for hundreds of millennia before we humans developed, and their DNA is very well adapted to adversity. They exist in large quantities and replicate exponentially at a great speed, and at each replication there is an opportunity to adapt. The progeny of the few survivors of an antibiotic attack will often partially and sometimes totally survive a repeated assault by the same antibiotic.

In the 1940s after the first antibiotics were developed, a wave of optimism swept through the medical profession. Everybody thought that all we needed to do was develop the right antibiotic for any specific bacterium and we would conquer infectious diseases. This has not come true at all. Nowadays we know that bacteria are the only creatures that truly prey on us, together with their cousins the viruses, prions, and other scary pieces of DNA. With just a little cynicism one could say that we are inadvertently helping bacteria and their ilk to become better and better at foiling our attempts to control them. The pharmaceutical companies nonetheless keep developing new and "better" antibiotics while resistance to existing antibiotics has become the latest medical nightmare.

So here were my thoughts as I was faced with one more bout of cystitis: Several times now I had narrowly followed the race of heroic inventions of more and more potent antibiotics just to heal a little cystitis, with only temporary results. I did get rid of the problem every time. It returned a few months later, though, as soon as I exposed myself to fatigue and dehydration. What if I caught a serious infection one day and the top-of-the-line antibiotic, which I recently used against a few new-generation *E. coli* thugs, would not help me at all?

This time I decided to follow rigorously the old-fashioned herbal cures that I had heard about. I mustered my courage, followed my own advice, and ingested massive amounts of antioxidant vitamins, herbs, cranberries, blueberries, and uva ursi as juices, capsules, extracts, and essences. Herbalists teach us that these substances eliminate *E. coli* bacteria from our bladder. Before antibiotics were invented, rest, heated compresses, herb teas, and fruit extracts used to be the only possible course of action to take in case of urinary tract infections, and our ancestors (or shall we call them "foremothers"?) took a long time to heal from cystitis, but they did survive, didn't they? I was successful too! Daily I swallowed large amounts of unsweetened cranberry concentrate, antioxidants like unbuffered vitamin C, herbal preparations like marine pine bark extract and grapefruit seed extract, and gallons of water. It took me only about ten days of that draconian regime to get rid of all symptoms like pain and urgency, but it took me three to four months until I did not have any more *E. coli* in my urine when I had it tested in the lab—and I continued using the herbs for all that time.

That is a very long time, too long for most of us, and it could be risky. The infection could rise into the kidneys if it gets out of hand. A further risk is that the bacteria that hurt you may not even be *E. coli.* If you try this I advise high dosages of all of the substances listed above and at least three quarts of water a day. Truly! If the herbal remedies produce nothing but an aggravation of the problem within a day or two, you must go to see your doctor as soon as possible!

Recently a better naturopathic way was found to eliminate the *E. coli* in the bladder without killing the *E. coli* in the large intestine. The substance contained in the berries that the herbalists recommend has been isolated and found to be a simple one-molecule sugar called mannose.[11] It is easy to understand that a simple crystallized sugar is more concentrated than berries or juice. Mannose turns out to be the chiral copy of glucose, the basic sugar that is the fuel for our bodies. A chiral copy is a mirror image where right and left are reversed, the same way the back of your right hand is like the back of your left hand (*chiro* is a Greek root word for "hand"). In other words, the substance is almost glucose but it is slightly screwy, with its molecular subgroups in the "wrong" spots. Therefore it is not useful to our physiology. If we drink water with mannose the digestive system uses very little of it; it discards most of the mannose right away from high up in the digestive tract, and it is excreted via the kidneys and the bladder—where it meets the *E. coli* bacteria. This is a very auspicious meeting: *E. coli* by far prefer mannose to the cells of a bladder wall. For them mannose is fast food. Mannose and *E. coli* unite and ride off into the sunset during urination. •Drink a glass of water containing one or two teaspoons of mannose eight to ten times a day for a while. End of the bladder infection, and no fallout for the colon!

The orthomolecular physician who drew my attention to this has cured chronically recurring bladder infections and dangerous kidney infections with mannose, a simple sugar. Let me insist on a very important point for us regarding this way (or the herbal and vitamin variety) of treating an *E. coli* infection of the bladder: the *E. coli* in the large intestine remain untouched and continue doing their beneficial work, furthering the digestion of complex molecules like amylopectins. It would be wise to continue drinking two to three quarts of water a day with mannose until you feel completely well, which means no pain nor heat with urination, clear and lightly colored urine, and, ideally, a negative lab test. I hope you are realizing, as we go along, that adding mannose to drinking water and consuming a large glass of it after intercourse would help clear the place of potential raptors. But, I repeat, if you are treating yourself with herbs and vitamins or mannose and you do not feel even a little better within a day or two after having started your treatment, you must call your doctor right away. Your problem may be too advanced, you may not have an *E. coli* infection, or you may be hosting more than one bacterium.

Are you still with me? We are not as far off track as it may seem. We are returning now to the common fluid retention not caused by hormonal imbalance but by intestinal trouble. Let us suppose, that, not knowing what I just told you about these stealthy ways of eliminating *E. coli* bacteria from your bladder, you have freed yourself from an *E. coli* urinary tract infection (or any other infection) with antibiotics, and you have proceeded to go back to your daily activities without restoring the normal flora in the large intestine.

A first risk to this approach is that the treatment may not have eliminated all the pathogenic bacteria, and your immune system may soon not be able to handle the survivors. Urinary infections recur frequently.

A second risk to this approach results from the misconception that after an antibiotic treatment there are no bacteria in the colon for a while. There are others, those that do not cause infections and those that were not sensitive to the large-spectrum antibiotic. As we have seen above, we live with bacteria; all kinds of them enter our digestive tract with food and many of them do survive digestion. If there are no *E. coli* or other beneficial bacteria present to defend the territory and to create the milieu needed, others will take over, multiply, settle in, and consume our food. Nothing will be noticed for a long time. In the meantime they will flourish, multiply, and spread to all parts of the intestine. They will find the amylopectins, the slow-digesting and partially undigested carbohydrates. This is real food for them. They will thrive with it. They will release gas and their own by-products of digestion, which are toxins to us.

The toxins released by the bacteria that are not normally present in our intestine, or at least not in large uncontrolled amounts, irritate the mucous membrane that lines the inner surface of the digestive tube. This membrane then releases abnormally large amounts of mucus to protect itself. The intestine is very discriminating; it will try not to allow any toxins to be absorbed into the bloodstream. This emergency procedure will, however, stop normal physiology. The regular exchange of fluids and nutritional substances moving through the capillaries of the intestinal walls will not happen. The consequences are increasing fluid retention inside the body and poor absorption of nutrition through the intestinal walls. Inside the intestinal tube there will be an accumulation of gas. In short, the invaders have won. The intestine has closed off its walls to protect the inside of the fortress, and the Huns are laying siege to the fields. They eat your food and they are having a great party at your expense. On top of that they reproduce like rabbits, have lousy manners, and fart a lot.

Tolerating the presence of such unwelcome hordes camping in the intestines will create the situation described above: feeling bloated after eating and being pestered by a very slow digestion. A late dinner becomes a reason for insomnia, the belly remains full and does not change for hours, gas pains linger, and malnutrition is a long-term consequence. Technically this is called dysbiosis. Constipation will slowly develop and, with time, the sufferer may end up taking laxatives. Laxatives are habit-forming and they are not a good solution, since they just force the intestines to empty. The person concerned will thus have given up any possibility for returning to a normal digestion.

I rarely read women's magazines, except when I am at the

hairdresser's or the dentist's. One day, turning pages sleepily, I noticed all the ads for "smooth relief" in the last pages of the magazines. I checked many other magazines for a while. Those ads are there all the time. This problem must be very common.

So what should be done? It may be difficult to have a doctor establish that colon bacteria are abnormal. Some of the bacteria involved are not even considered pathogens. So could a doctor even prescribe an antibiotic? Which antibiotic would that be? And what could be the possible use of nuking the invaders again anyway? As soon as the dust has settled, some of the pesky critters will have survived, their offspring will have mutated, other cousins will have infiltrated themselves under the cover of incoming food, and the colony will continue to proliferate.

It looks as though nothing will prevent this situation from persisting for a long time because we had to almost totally sacrifice the colon cops, our commensal bacteria buddies, the *E. coli* and other controlling species in our intestines, with antibiotics to save the bladder. In the present situation there is only one clever strategy. We have to embargo their food deliveries and radically starve them! We know what these unwelcome bacteria want: they want starch, they want the amylopectins that are not fully digested. We have to completely stop eating them for a while. It will take time and focus, but it will work. In cases of minor peripheral fluid retention and abdominal distress, the problem can be solved in a matter of weeks. Gradually digestion will become easier, the abdomen will not be swollen anymore, nor will there be excessive gas, and the transit will last only a day or so. It can take some more time on the diet until the bacterial balance has been re-established. Adding acidophilus and other probiotics to the diet for many months is a must.

The starches or carbohydrates that have to be systematically ignored are found in any and all grains—including rye, millet, and buckwheat—and all things made with grains. Then, to expedite the process we also need to eliminate white sugar and any other sugars like fructose, maltose, and lactose (yes, milk too, but not dry fermented cheese, since the fermentation transforms the sugar). These sugars need digestion and would be found and eaten by the bacteria. Also, of course, no breakfast cereals, cake, chocolate, bread, corn, potatoes, sweet potatoes, or rice. This process is difficult to start. I used the phrase "systematically ignored" on purpose. We need to talk to our higher selves about this! For us those starches have become most inferior food, causing gas and swelling in the belly. Off with their heads! Starches from any other vegetables, squashes, and fruit have simpler structures and will be successfully digested. A diet of moderate amounts of good-quality protein like organically raised meat and eggs, fish, pre-soaked beans, plenty of seasonal vegetables, vegetable oils, fresh fruits, dry cheese, and nuts will work. If a sweet is absolutely necessary, have some raw honey—it's mostly glucose. Some stores carry powdered glucose.

If you have the intestinal woes described above and you spend a few weeks or months on such a diet, you will probably discover that your intestines are functioning much easier, that your abdomen is not causing you trouble anymore, and that you have lost weight without going hungry. As you feel better and you slowly reintroduce sugar and refined flour, pasta, fries, and cake into your diet, you may feel fine.[12]

You may also not really like what these starches do for you anymore. Soon after they have left your taste buds and start being digested, you may observe that they make you feel heavy, that your digestion is slower, and that "post-prandial torpor"—the goofy tiredness that comes over you after having eaten a heavy meal or a monster dessert—is seriously cramping your style!

Here I am leaving the topic of poor digestion and fluid retention caused by the presence of abnormal bacterial flora in the intestines to make a little tangent toward nutrition as it relates to proprioception, the art of perceiving one's internal sensations. If you do not like the way the amylopectin starches make you feel, why eat them at all? Many people belong among the descendants of hunters and gatherers, not agriculturists. As a result, they do not naturally have an enzyme system that allows them to feel well after eating dense amylopectin starches. These foods are called "comfort foods" by the people who like them. Well, for you, they are discomfort foods! The Christians among us pray for bread in the Lord's Prayer. That is understandable. There were famines in past centuries where bread was the only food around because grains could be stored. But now that you can perceive the cause of your discomfort, and you do not live in a country where there is a serious lack of food (at least I very much hope you don't), focus on what you really like to eat. I love the smell of fresh bread. I mostly do not touch it. After years of not eating bread I had a bite of it one day. My husband asked me, "So, what is it like?" I sat there chewing and answered, "Like eating very nice-tasting cardboard." In the same vein, I love the smell of my perfume. It would not occur to me to drink it.

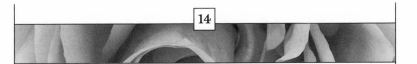

hot flashes

HOT FLASHES ARE not necessarily a sign of the onset of meno-pause; they are a symptom of very low estrogen. Hot flashes happen to young women who have low estrogen; they also may have very low body fat from dieting or from over-exercising. If this is the case for a young woman, she needs to attend to it if she wants to be healthy and fertile. On the other hand, if hot flashes happen to a woman in her late forties or early fifties, it is reasonable to think, of course, that the peri-menopausal phase has started.

As we have seen, premenstrual syndrome is related to estrogen excess and to progesterone deficiency. When peri-menopausal hot flashes occur, the picture changes. Progesterone is the first hormone to really diminish and eventually disappear almost completely. It is the decrease of estrogen and hormones related to the release of the ovum from the ovary, however, that is generally thought of as the real beginning of menopause and the cause for hot flashes. Even after menopause the ovaries still make some estrogen, but much less. The body will never be completely without estrogen, because estrogen is made not only by the ovaries, but also by the adrenals. This hormone has many important functions throughout all of life for both women and men. During menopause most of the production of estrogen is supposed to move from the ovaries to the adrenal glands.

What are hot flashes? The first one might be creepy: A strange sensation starts, one that you have never felt, if you are attentive.

It may resemble the cold sweat you might have felt if you had suddenly faced a mortal danger—for example, if you had just escaped being creamed in traffic by a big truck, except there is nothing of that sort going on. You might be just minding your normal everyday business. If the hot flash happens in the middle of the night you might first suddenly be wide awake for no perceivable reason, then feel very hot and begin to sweat on your back, neck, or torso.

There is no end of war stories about extreme hot flashes. They can cause high anxiety, severe dehydration, and disabling insomnia. They can soak nice business outfits in minutes and leave sufferers with red-hot faces. One woman I know in Europe who suffered from severe hot flashes said her doctor tested her level of dehydration by making her hold a piece of sugar under her tongue. He measured the time it took for the sugar to dissolve. She said she sat there for half an hour with the sugar barely changed. When I was in high school I observed my overweight history teacher talking at length about the pharaoh Amenhotep IV. She would turn beet-red, and sweat would run down her full-moon face. She would remain totally unfazed, get her hanky, mop her face, and ask us to open all the windows in the middle of a snowstorm. I never understood why Amenhotep IV had that strange effect on her.

Hot flashes are considered normal. Here, again, we have to ask: What does "normal" mean? Average? Usual? Common? Considering that some of us sail through menopause with a few night sweats and not much else, I dare say that if hot flashes become a major pain in the unmentionable, they have nothing to do with "normal" and they need to be managed. They indicate a severe hormonal imbalance. The dehydration alone is not conducive to the health of the body; the anxiety and the embarrassment hot flashes can cause are catastrophic to the mind. I know a woman who cancelled her social life, thinking she had become a bother to her friends. Any good health practitioner will agree to treat this condition, and drastically differing therapies are offered with a great range of efficiency.

In short, if a woman's hot flashes are totally disruptive, happen all the time, soak clothes and sheets, and prevent sleep, then she needs to seek outside help. I advise the same routes as for other consequences of hormonal imbalance: acupuncture, homeopathy, herbs. It might even be a good idea to combine some of these approaches before considering bio-identical hormone supplementation. Ask around and find an experienced practitioner. The simple addition of hormones to the system will have wide-reaching side effects, and those who take hormones need regular monitoring. As I said earlier, during menopause the body is switching most of the production of estrogen from the ovaries to the adrenal glands. Taking estrogen, even bio-identical estrogen, will not help the body make that transition—it will delay it. Some of what women with extreme menopausal symptoms experience may not be due only to menopause; they may also be suffering from pre-existing adrenal exhaustion or latent thyroid problems. The careful approach is always the same: minimize side effects and avoid major changes that are induced when chemical substances that are foreign to the body are used.

To all of those women with milder symptoms, a friendly wake-up call: Don't shrink away, stay here! What is happening? Aren't you soon going to be liberated from the so-called curse? Aren't you looking forward to freedom from the ever-recurring monthly rise and fall of body and mind, which needs endless, boring management, planning, and patience? So let's imagine that we are going to find help, learn how to minimize excessive symptoms, and ride the wave smoothly. Mild hot flashes can be fun, even attractive. You suddenly take your sweater and your shirt off, and spend some time in your tank top in the middle of action, then put them back on soon after. Real lovers like that—they are into sweet sweat! You may grow to like it, too: it keeps you very awake. Just incorporate hot flashes into your day. After the heat wave comes a very nice little cool moment when the sweat evaporates. Dress in appropriate layers!

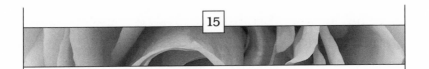

insomnia

THERE ARE SO many kinds of insomnia! If you are one of the many people who suffer from sleeplessness (insomnia is a Latin word for no *somnus* or sleep), ask yourself: Why can't you sleep? What is the nature of the obstacle? Does it affect your body? Does it affect your mind? Just hanging out for month after month and waiting for insomnia to go away by itself is a very bad strategy. Deep sleep is a necessity. Short naps during the day are no replacement for deep REM (rapid eye movement) sleep, the integrative sleep that includes dreaming. One major physiological process that happens during deep sleep is the release of growth hormone from the pituitary gland. Human Growth Hormone is a precursor to all other hormone release. Menopause-induced insomnia is a sign that your body has a hard time with the transition. But insomnia is not necessarily just a menopausal problem. It can happen to people who have trouble managing their energy and people who gradually have taken on habits that affect sleep, like heavy and long-term consumption of alcohol and/or coffee.

The long-term consequences of sleep deprivation are insidious and cumulative. They affect you deeply by making you physically and emotionally more and more fragile. The absence of dreaming affects your psyche, by preventing your unconscious from expressing itself, so to speak. Insomnia also compromises your immune system; any rampant bug may catch you if you are deeply fatigued. Remember that sleep deprivation is also a very efficient method of torture—it breaks the spirit of political prisoners and drives them insane.

You may be inclined to "solve" the problem with sleeping pills. Sleeping pills are, so to speak, generic sleep inducers. Insomnia carries an important message. You are not a generic person and you should not be contented with a generic weapon to kill the messenger.

If you look up any sleeping pill in the *Physician's Desk Reference* you will see that it is considered a psychiatric medication. Don't let your MD or gynecologist prescribe psychiatric medication to you. It is beyond their scope of practice. Like any psychiatric medication, sleeping pills have side effects. You will see that long-term use can damage liver and kidney function, and there is a strong likelihood that they cause personality changes, including severe depression.[13] As with many psychiatric medications, sleeping pills are designed for temporary use only. You also will read that physician supervision is necessary. Many people are very happy with their sleeping pills. They do not check in with their doctor for many months and they request refills via their pharmacist. Where is the safety check? I may appear unreasonably alarmist, but I know for a fact that almost all the lost young people—the high school and university students who take up arms and kill others and themselves in their schools—were on psychiatric medication. Look up the reporting; somewhere you will find it mentioned.

If medication for insomnia is needed, it must be accompanied by a therapeutic relationship with a psychiatrist who is familiar with this very delicate condition. Good psychiatrists exist—find them via referrals from your MD or from friends you trust. Do not stay with a doctor who simply prescribes for you without demanding that you check in with her or him. Avoid buying multiple refills, which your doctor may allow without seeing you first.

Sleep inducers from the alternative medicine world like mela-tonin, which is a hormone, or 5HTP (5 Hydroxytryptophan), which is made with the amino acid tryptophan, and a great variety of calming herbs like valerian or chamomile, alone or in varying combinations, should also be considered a temporary help only. Do not rely on them. Not sleeping is a message. Don't offend your intelligence, if I dare say so. You will be able to figure out what you need.

So let's leave the potentially dangerous route for now and see if we can come up with some creative approaches to insomnia. Shouldn't we always first try the least damaging approach?

If you cannot stop thinking about actual serious inner or outer conflicts affecting your life, you may need to seek outside psychological help from a therapist or a Neuro-Linguistic Programmer who can set things into a manageable context.

Maybe your body is bone-tired but your mind keeps racing in a rather absurd way. Why is that so? Perhaps you did some-thing fitting any of the following categories shortly before lying down: Have you thought incessantly about solving a complicated task? Have you watched a very exciting shoot-'em-up movie? Have you driven one hundred miles on the freeway at breakneck speed? Have you had a screaming argument with somebody close to you? Have you played a war video game? In brief, did you spend time in emergency mode? If so, your sympathetic nervous system has been engaged and now at bedtime you are lying there spinning your wheels.

Get up and get a book. Read something that talks to you about growing orchids or visiting the ruins of Macchu Picchu, about how your town looked in 1870, about the achievements of the munchkins in the local Steiner school, or an award given to a ninety-year-old music teacher. Understand that you need to exit emergency mode and identify with something pretty that makes you feel at peace and might induce lovely yawns. It may take some time, but it will happen. Just persist. You may sleep only a few hours that night. The better approach would be to plan your schedule so that you avoid entering emergency mode in the evening. You may think that your life does not permit this right now. But it really is your choice whether you race your mind around until late at night or slow down to get ready for sleep.

Perhaps you consumed more coffee or stronger coffee than you normally drink? Did you drink an herb tea that contained green tea? Did you drink white wine? Did you eat chocolate with caffeine in it? If yes, you are out of luck—the problem is not in your mind. Get up and work on your taxes. The substances you enjoyed will keep you awake until they have made it out of your system. Think about why or how you were lured into making the mistake.

Is your skin so sensitive that your favorite sheets are scratchy? Are your legs twitchy? Is there just no comfortable spot nor position to be found in bed? Do you hear every airplane, truck, cat, or owl? Is your peacefully and quietly sleeping sweetheart breathing too loud? Is that the electricity coursing through the walls or are your ears ringing?

Here too, find the remedy that is at the level of the problem. In this case it will help to take a hot bath or a long hot shower. Use up the entire water tank: no one else will need hot water at two in the morning. Stay in there, hum a song to yourself. Take a fashion magazine with you if you sit in the tub. By heating your skin, you will push the hypersensitivity up and over the edge and it will turn itself off.

There are at least two good reasons why this technique works. The first has to do with the tenth cranial nerve, the vagus nerve, which wanders out of the head, down the neck, along the lungs and the heart, and into the upper digestive system. This nerve is part of the cranial nerves, which manage the parasympathetic nervous system, the life-supporting functions that induce peristaltic motion for digestion, regulate breathing and heart beat, and govern relaxation and sleep. Heating the neck, the upper thorax, and the abdomen will induce relaxation for this reason. The other good reason relates to the cranio-sacral rhythm, the rhythm inherent in the support system that holds your brain and spinal cord in place. Lying in the tub and really abandoning your head against its hard edge can equilibrate your cranio-sacral rhythm. Dr. William Garner Sutherland, one of the venerable old osteopaths and the father of cranial osteopathy, learned about this by observing himself as he rested his head on a hard surface.

If you cannot use hot water, do something with your muscles. Very slow yoga stretches can help. There are actually specific yoga stretches for sleep: look them up. Taking a short walk out into the night or hanging out at your window or in the garden looking at the moon could help too.

The royal route for disconnecting from daily preoccupations and stresses, however, is meditation. If you are experiencing insomnia, now may be a very good time to start learning how to meditate, or to go back to your practice, or to have a meeting with your teacher, or to seek a teacher who is beloved and recommended by a friend. Don't you go out now and tell everybody that I advise meditation to cure insomnia! One of my teachers called the passing-out that happened to me in the early stages of learning meditation, "stupid meditation."

"It is very good for you," he said, "it makes your body relax. But," he added with an impish smile, "it does nothing in the direction of your enlightenment."

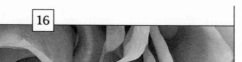

anxiety

What does it avail you to attribute
to the happenings in life the cause of misery
which is really within you?
—RAMANA MAHARSHI

NAMING AN OUTSIDE cause for an inner state is a common mistake among us neurotics. "There must be a reason for how I feel," we think, and if we search around long enough we will find one. For those among us who have learned to notice the global shift that happened with ovulation when we were still fertile, menopause can become more manageable. We know that we are the ones who have changed, and if the change can be understood, a possibility for returning to homeostasis can be found, even though it will be a different homeostasis.

It is easy to recognize physical changes. Many of us are quite focused on our appearance, since we have been led to understand that it is one of our essential assets and our best tool of manipulation. So, in the face of adversities like swelling or weight gain, we wear loose clothes, work out more, eat less, get advice from the naturopaths or the medical doctors, take vitamins, drugs, or herbs—anything to hide, manage, or get rid of the unwelcome temporary change.

The difficult part is recognizing psychological hypersensitivity, even if it sets on rather suddenly. Yes, your beloved might really have said something borderline insensitive, selfish, or housedragon-like, and yes, it hurts. Had you been in a post-menstrual state, you might have said or at least thought, "Must be tough to live in your shoes too!" But in an anxious state you can't do that. You impute evil intentions to the poor wretch while he or she just innocently bumbles through the day managing his or her own frustrations. If your darling is a man, and hence almost certainly someone who has no experience with cyclic hormonal vicissitudes, you may be facing a long pouting and counter-pouting period. Let's not forget that most men simply do not have the luck to have perceivable symptoms of their own hormone shifts. They are subjected to them though, and they might project their troubles on us and think that we too are brutal and selfish.

If menopause approaches in a milieu of previously well established hormonal imbalance, its psychological aspects can become really nasty. One such event is the true anxiety attack, a problem known in the emergency rooms. The patient may have a resting pulse rate rising up to 140 beats per minute, an ominous feeling that a catastrophe is about to happen or already happening, intense sweating, and an ugly fear of having a heart attack. How could this possibly be psychological? Well, it is not entirely psychological, of course. People experiencing these symptoms often feel scared enough to call the ambulance. The paramedics, seeing someone freaked out, generally give them oxygen to lower the pulse rate and want to take them to the emergency room. If the paramedics are well trained, their thinking is: If she is scared enough to call us, she should be checked. Of course, the electro-cardiogram and lab tests would reveal that everything is just fine. The ensuing diagnosis of "anxiety attack" would seem to be such an insult. If the patient is lucky, someone will explain that she is not hysterical, and that anxiety attacks can happen to anyone in a stressful situation. (Literally all women are hysterical, since *hysterion* means "uterus" in ancient Greek, but I will spare you the

digression into the unfortunate historical origins of this word.)
Even those who don't experience true dramatic anxiety attacks
may still become more anxious during menopause. Things that
were uncomfortable before may now become disabling and
may develop into real phobias like fears of heights or water, or
going on airplanes or to the bank machine at night. My sweet
grandmother was afraid of ugly bearded guys out there in the
bushes at night. She shut and locked all doors, closed all shutters
and all windows as soon as the sun set. My mother did not even
consider going to the underground parking lot of her apartment
building at night. Fears of this type can become disabling enough
to warrant psychiatric care.

Aside from psychiatric methods, there are alternative
approaches to treating anxiety. An osteopath with whom I discussed the symptoms of hormone imbalance stated with certainty
that anxiety is due to a cranial problem. Needless to say, he
practiced cranial osteopathy. I am not implying that the man was
wrong; there are many aspects to any health issue. He sounded
convincing as he said, "If the pressure on your pituitary gland
is not released you will think that outside events are oppressive
to you." It might be useful to know that the pituitary gland, also
called the "master gland," releases precursory hormones that
govern most hormonal changes, including fluid retention.

Acupuncture is another avenue to explore in treating anxiety,
in part because acupuncture has a very interesting view of the
mind-body connection. Experienced practitioners recognize
emotions as part and parcel of disturbances in the circulation
of vital energy (called "chi"). For example, having a short fuse is
due to liver meridian trouble; feeling despair is kidney meridian
trouble, etc. The teaching is complex and profound. Those who
are skeptical about acupuncture probably know strictly nothing about it, or may have met only incompetent practitioners.
Consider the benefits that acupuncture can bring to you. Three

thousand years of collective thinking and clinical experience cannot possibly be all wrong!

I have the same thing to say about unmanageable anxiety as I said about unmanageable insomnia: try the best alternative practitioners before you consider psychiatric medication. If you do take medication, remain in contact with your doctor. Never forget that synthetic medication very often is damaging to the liver or to the kidneys or to both. We know that the unwelcome symptoms of menopause are due to a problematic hormone physiology. We also know that the liver is the organ that "catabolizes," that cuts up large hormone molecules and prepares them for elimination. (It performs at least two hundred other life-maintaining tasks.) Likewise, the kidneys are very specific filtering organs: they simultaneously filter out into the urine what we do not need and reabsorb what we do need back into the bloodstream. Taking into account that the liver and kidneys are our most important detoxification organs, it is clear that using medication that will heavily tax these organs is only to be considered if all else has failed.

the pesky "why" question

*Do not believe anything merely because it is said, nor
in the traditions because they have been handed down
from antiquity, nor in rumors as such, nor in writings by
sages because sages wrote them, nor in fancies that
we may suspect to have been inspired in us by a deva, nor
in inferences drawn from some haphazard assumption we
may have made, nor in what seems to be an analogical
necessity, nor in the mere authority of our teachers
and masters. Believe when the writing, doctrine or saying
is corroborated by reason and consciousness.*

—Prince Siddhartha Gautama,
the Buddha, 563–483 BC

THE SAYING GOES that while religion evolves from truth to truth, science goes from error to error. It is probable that fifty percent of what I told you above is wrong already, and I cannot tell you now which is the wrong part. Only time will tell. I also simplified many things to make them easily understandable, thereby risking imprecision and the scorn of the learned. All I can say about that is: I'm trembling already. If you find out that some of my errors have been discovered in the meantime, please let me know.

The purpose of my writing was to take away creepy fears about our bodies. My greatest hope is to have shown you how to think about what you feel and how to find help when you think you need it, how to look for a sympathetic and even compassionate connection with the people you choose for help, and, above all, to never let anybody convince you that you are okay when you don't feel okay.

It is a good thing to have a doctor or an alternative practitioner who knows you, a person you trust, a person with whom you can have a so-called therapeutic relationship. It is more conventional to have a therapeutic relationship with a psychotherapist. But I think it is also good to look for one with people who attend to your body, because, frankly, I have come to think that we can't possibly decide that there is such a clear difference. I concluded this the day I learned about the physical problems of psychiatric patients who are diagnosed with Multiple Personality Disorder (now called Dissociative Identity Disorder). It has been observed that the two different personalities can have very different physiological characteristics and even different health problems. One could have high blood pressure, the other one low blood pressure. I could handle that example: our inner state can alter our blood pressure. Then I learned that one personality could have diabetes, and not the other.[14] There I stalled. It stretched me beyond my possibilities to be asked to believe that diabetes is a psychosomatic problem—unless we agree that all problems are more or less psychosomatic. I am not at all ready to go there. In great confusion I asked one of my teachers, "So who am I, my body or my mind?" He said, "You are the one who notices."

As for those of us who practice manual medicine, it is impossible, in my opinion, not to have a therapeutic relationship with people we take care of by touching them continuously for an hour or longer. It is also common practice for Rolfers, osteopaths, chiropractors, and many other manipulative therapists to see people over a long period of time. We practitioners generally agree that we help people heal or recover or develop their body, their only tool of self-expression. The patients may or may not be aware of how much we are involved with each other, and that is okay with me.

I mentioned above that in a therapeutic relationship one

should look for sympathy and compassion. That's at least what I would do if I were looking for help. I would feel better if I thought that I had an insight into the nature of the person I had chosen to help me. But not everybody is the lovey-dovey type. A dear friend of mine from Europe had a dangerous lymphoma and was treated with chemotherapy. I spoke to him on the telephone whenever I could reach him. I was very concerned for him and inquired if his oncologist knew him, and also if his doctor spoke to him about himself and his medical approach to the disease. My friend told me that it was not in the least important to him that his oncologist knew anything about him nor that he knew anything about his oncologist. The only thing that needed to be known was the diagnosis, the lab values, and their evolution as the treatment proceeded. He said that from his point of view doctors should stick to their work and not try to "rub up" on patients, that it would make them look goofy and in need of being liked. I saw his point.

Let's look at an alternate example: A friend of mine, who is an MD and a homeopath, told me about one of her first experiences as a homeopath. A woman came to see her complaining of long-term and intractable constipation. My friend took the case and found it very complex. She prescribed a remedy. Two weeks later the woman came back beaming, so happy to have found such a marvelous doctor. She told my friend that the medicine had made her feel so good, and that she had not felt that good for such a long time; and she had come back to consult about her constipation, which had not changed at all.

Disease and healing are never simple. All is always connected to who we are, to what we do, to what we believe, to our inherited organ weaknesses, etc., and there can be very different successful approaches to the same problem. I have a coffee table book in my waiting room titled *Spontaneous Remissions*.[15] It tells about people who heal from correctly diagnosed serious illnesses, mostly cancers, which are considered irremediably fatal by everybody who has a medical education. There is no scientific explanation for the spontaneous remissions. The doctors speak about the "spectrum of Self-Repair." Psycho-neuro-immunology is brought forth. But the medical professionals have trouble even agreeing on what a spontaneous remission is. Did the remission really not have a cause, or were they just not able to see it? Meanwhile, the surviving patients attribute their healing to an interesting array of causes: prayer, meditation and hypnosis, exposure to hot air and baths, diet changes and alternative therapies, changes of occupation, changes of residence, long journeys, strong will to live, raging against one's fate, and simple denial. This book includes descriptions of very unusual and even potentially heretical medical procedures that apparently brought about remissions. A first example: blood transfusions, the blood being taken from people who survived the same cancer. A second example: inoculation with an active infection to rally the immune system, based on the observation that some dangerous cancers have disappeared after a serious and unrelated inflammatory disease has healed.

Generally the book's authors agree that the diseases happened in the first place because the patients' immune systems were compromised due to age-related genetic damage and to physical and psychological responses to extreme stress. They also agree that the healing must have occurred because the immune system rallied to the task anyway. This book is very descriptive of how baffled conventional doctors can be when faced with the fact that things can work out for patients who are in deep trouble; the specialists act almost as if it is not right that a predicted fatal outcome should not happen.

If you peruse the alternative medicine journals published by a great variety of groups of conventionally trained doctors who work on the margins or progressive edge of mainstream science, or very modern-thinking people trained in the medical traditions of India and China, you will see that there is no end of really bright people who have bright ideas, and that there are even more bright people who combine other bright people's bright ideas into consistently bright theories about why things happen in healing and disease. The publications are full of this. Let's welcome all bright ideas. But they are all worthless nonsense if they are not accompanied by extensive clinical experience and years of repeated confirmation of results, no matter the school of thinking to which the doctors belong. Every honest doctor or healer will tell you, however, that consistent results may not necessarily provide us with a sound scientific explanation about why something is successful, which is certainly no reason to not keep looking.

notes

1. In 2003 the number of women diagnosed with breast cancer dropped by 7% (*The Wall Street Journal*, December 15, 2006). Doctors assumed it happened because women stopped taking artificial hormones and took more calcium and more anti-inflammatory drugs. On the same day, *The New York Times* published a front-page article saying that a common form of women's breast cancer dropped 15% from August 2002 to December 2003 and that all types of breast cancer dropped 7%.

   On January 11, 2007, an article in the *Wall Street Journal*, "The Hormone Decision: How to Weigh the Risks," detailed extensively the risks of artificial hormone supplementation.

2. The Nurses' Health Study, 1976, indicated that hormone therapy benefits women with menopausal problems. (121,700 registered female nurses participated.) A second very large study, The Women's Health Initiative, the largest randomized controlled clinical trial of hormone treatment carried out by the National Institutes of Health, was halted in 2002 when researchers concluded that hormone supplementation increased the risks of breast cancer, stroke and blood clots, and that there was no protection from heart disease.

3. The "Skindeep" website is an excellent resource to check out cosmetics, www.cosmeticsdatabase.com.

4. A detailed article about pelvic pain can be found in the *Townsend Letter* of November 2006, page 72, by Tori Hudson, ND, "Chronic Pelvic Pain, Part I, Prevalence, Etiology, Diagnosis."

5. Mammograms are very difficult and tiring to read. Radiologists read many in a day. Sometimes they simply may not see a problem; sometimes they change their mind about what they see. If shown a mammogram they had evaluated and classified as presenting a potential cancer some time earlier, they may not see the same problem when looking at it a second time. All mammograms should always be read separately by two people. This is not done routinely. More information about diagnostic imaging can be found

in Chapter 8, "The Eye of the Beholder," of Dr. Jerome Groopman's book *How Doctors Think* (New York: Houghton Mifflin, 2007).

6. See Chapter 8, "The Eye of the Beholder," in *How Doctors Think* by Jerome Groopman, MD (New York: Houghton Mifflin, 2007).

7. To learn about uterine fibroids in detail, see Paul Indman, MD's website: www.hopeforfibroids.org. To learn more about risk factors and an alternative to surgery for uterine fibroids, read the *Townsend Letter*, November 2006, "Phytotherapy for Uterine Fibroids," page 64, Kerry Bone, www.mediherb.com.

8. Alice Waters, grande dame of the California Nouvelle Cuisine movement, has published a series of great cooking books.

9. The many different names for sugar that you can find on labels include: fructose, corn syrup, high fructose corn syrup, brown rice syrup, malt syrup, refiner's syrup, sorghum syrup, blackstrap molasses, molasses, apple juice and/or grape juice concentrate, cane juice, dextran, dextrose, invert sugar, lactose, maltose, maltodextrin, mannitol, sorbitol, sucrose, yellow sugar, etc. There are more: look for words ending in "ose" and "ol". Any syrup or anything related to molasses is sugar.

These sugars are not all the same, of course, but they are metabolized (digested and assimilated) in a similar way and end up as fat stored in your adipose cells. I am not opposed to sugar out of principle, if it is consumed in reasonable quantities. But look up the increase of sugar consumption in the last twenty years, correlate it with the increase of obesity and also correlate it with the increase of diabetes... and you will see why I had to stick this in here.

10. A book published in 1966, *Feminine Forever* by Dr. Robert A. Wilson (New York: M. Evans and Company, 1966), started the prescribing of estrogen for menopausal women. Jerome Groopman, MD, informs us in his book *How Doctors Think* (New York: Houghton Mifflin, 2007), page 210: "It turned out that a drug company that made estrogen had paid Dr. Wilson to write the book."

11. Search on the Internet for Dr. Jonathan V. Wright's article, "D-Mannose for Bladder and Kidney Infections."

12. The book *Breaking the Vicious Cycle* by Elaine Gottschall (Ontario, Canada: The Kirkton Press, 1994) addresses serious intestinal problems like Crohn's disease, ulcerative colitis, and chronic diarrhea. She explains how an appropriate diet can gradually reverse these serious diseases. The essential information here is that starches and sugars made of complex molecules will not be digested by a digestive system that does not operate optimally.

Most recent information is based on this understanding. Gottschall also gives us ways to think about changing habitual eating, how to replace our staples with different foods, etc.

13. The book *Darkness Visible: A Memoir of Madness* by William Styron (New York: Random House, 1990) is not about insomnia *per se*. It is about depression. It is a compelling description of the downward spiraling of a great mind and its lucky return. We are brought to understand that, in his case, excesses of alcohol consumption combined with excessive doses of sleeping pills brought him to the edge of suicide.

14. A mention about diabetes in patients with Multiple Personality Disorder can be found in: *Frontier Perspectives*. Vol. 15, Number 1, Spring/Summer 2006, pp. 32–39. See "The Rehabilitation Potential of the Diabetic" by Stephen Patascher, PhD. Email: drpat@cox.net.

15. *Spontaneous Remissions: An Annotated Bibliography* is published by the Institute of Noetic Sciences, www.noetic.org/publications.cfm.

resources

A VERY GOOD resource for natural medicine, sustainable eco-
logical practices of all sorts, resources to find the doctor you
need, great articles about how to structure your home and
business in a "green" way, etc., can be found at Teleosis Institute,
teleosis.org.

NATUROPATHY

To find a naturopathic doctor: www.naturopathic.org, American
Association of Naturopathic Physicians.

THE IMAGING OF BREAST TISSUE

Informative books: *Preventing Breast Cancer,* Jon W. Gofman, MD,
PhD (1996). C.N.R. Book Division, Committee for Nuclear
Responsibility, Inc., P.O. Box 421993, San Francisco, CA
94142.

The Breast Cancer Prevention Program, Dr. Samuel Epstein, MD, and
David Steinman with Suzanne LeVert (New York: Macmillan, A
Simon and Schuster Company, 1997).

To find Licensed Board-Certified Thermographers in the U.S.
call 866.766.2468.

In the San Francisco Bay Area, contact Nancy Gardner, PhD, at Optimum Health Clinic, Inc., 712 D Street, Suite L, San Rafael, CA 94901, 415.480.9722. For Dr. Gardner's classes on preventing breast cancer and mobile thermography screening locations, check her website at: www.healthybreasts.info under "Upcoming Events."

NUTRITION

To find a local farmer's market: www.localharvest.org.

To find local producers of sustainably raised meat, poultry, dairy, eggs: www.eatwellguide.org.

To find out how commercial meat is produced read *Modern Meat* (New York: Vintage Books, 1983) by Orville Schell, Faculty of UC Berkeley, Journalism Dept.

To learn about pesticides: www.foodnews.org.

For further information, see *The Safe Shopper's Bible* by David Steinman and Samuel S. Epstein, MD (Hoboken, NJ: Wiley, 1995).

To learn the principles of California Nouvelle Cuisine, read the books of Alice Waters. They can be found on amazon.com.

NEWSLETTERS WITH GENERAL INFORMATION

• The newsletter that I have been reading and liking for years is *Nutrition and Healing* by Jonathan V. Wright, MD. Dr. Wright is the director of the Tahoma Clinic in Renton, Washington. His monthly publication features invaluable information about prevention and healing with bio-identical hormones and other natural substances like vitamins, herbs, mushrooms, probiotics, and enzymes. He teaches about possible side effects of various combinations and high dosages.

Wright is also a very intense advocate for naturopathy, and he does not miss any opportunity to tell us how politics can and do interfere with naturopathy and how we can help, if we are so inclined.

He is usually the first one to report about new discoveries. He also reports on natural compounds that have been successfully used in the past but discarded and forgotten after medications deemed more efficacious, but often having deleterious side effects, were developed by pharmaceutical companies. He reports about other naturopathic doctors and their discoveries.

Dr. Wright can be irreverent, even incendiary. He will stand up for people who have been persecuted because of new discoveries that are very promising and even proven to be effective clinically. Have fun reading him! If one of my family members or friends were found to have a serious problem I would definitely ask for his insights. He lets us know where we can buy the substances he speaks about, and he also carries them in the dispensary of his clinic.

The Lark Letter: A Woman's Guide to Optimum Health and Balance is very good and informative, with sound, well-worded, and careful advice. The publication markets vitamins and supplements of the author's own design.

Magazines

* *Townsend Letter, The Examiner of Alternative Medicine* is a peer-reviewed medical monthly review containing much-needed technical information, regular columns, research reports, and book critiques about most topics of natural and alternative medicine, including naturopathy, homeopathy, acupuncture, and herbalism. For sale in all good health food stores.

▸*Alternative Medicine, The Art and Science of Healthy Living* is an "easy reading" and entertaining monthly magazine. It addresses most important health issues in a style that is clear and understandable for people who do not have a medical education. It definitely can encourage people to learn more about prevention and to start thinking about options if they have problems.

Websites and Email Addresses

service@HealthierNews.com—information about the *Nutrition and Healing* newsletter

www.naturopathic.org—American Association of Naturopathic Physicians

townsendletter.com

www.noetic.org/publications.cfm

Seminar

"The Heat Is On," a one-day, eight-hour seminar for women and professionals in the health care field, is the most thorough information on women's health you can get in one day. Dr. Lani Simpson has taught this seminar for years. She is very knowledgeable and clear and above all up to date on new research. Her website: lanisimpson.com.

index

about the author

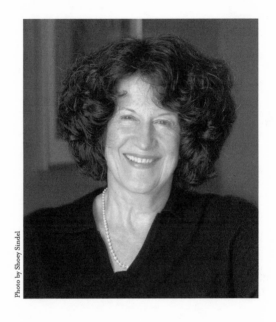

GEORGETTE MARIA DELVAUX, DC, was born in Luxembourg. Originally trained as a translator, she speaks five languages. She studied psychology in Geneva, Switzerland, and came to the United States to study Rolfing. She graduated from the Rolf Institute of Structural Integration in Boulder, Colorado, in 1979, and was certified as an Advanced Rolfer in 1986. A licensed chiropractor since 1992, Dr. Delvaux also practices craniosacral osteopathy and pursues her interest in nutritional science. She currently shares a Rolfing practice with her husband, Michael Salveson, in Berkeley, California, and in her spare time she likes to practice her cello.